LIVE LONGER AND STRONGER WITH BREAST CANCER

A Step-By-Step Guide

DR. LORI BOUCHARD, ND, BHSC
Copyright © **Lori Bouchard, 2020**

Published 2020

www.insidehealthclinic.com

Publishers Note: This is a work of non-fiction. Names have been changed for confidentiality purposes. Any resemblance to actual people, living or dead, or to businesses, companies, events, institutions, or locales is completely coincidental.

The information in this book is for educational purposes only. It is not intended to treat or diagnose illness. All health conditions should be reviewed by a qualified healthcare professional. You must inform your physician about any prescription drugs and supplements you are taking before changing. The author does not take any responsibility for individuals who choose to self-diagnose, self-treat or use the information in this book without consulting with their own healthcare practitioners.

Neither the author nor the publisher assumes any responsibility for errors, omissions, or contrary interpretations of the subject matter herein. Any perceived slight of any individual or organization is purely unintentional.

Brand and product names are trademarks or registered trademarks of their respective owners.

Live Longer and Stronger with Breast Cancer / Dr. Lori Bouchard – 1st edition.

ISBN: 9798555955449
Imprint: Independently published

ADVANCED PRAISE

"Few things can rock a person's world like the words 'You have cancer.'" Few things leave one with more of a need for support, information, guidance and love. Dr Lori Bouchard delivers all four in a stunningly simple arrangement of complex data, leaving an overwhelmed person feeling what they most want to feel at a time of fear and despair: a sense of hope. May this book fall into the hands of everyone who needs it, for it will definitely lighten the burden on both their body and their soul."

- Marianne Williamson, NY Times Best Selling Author 'A Return to Love'

"It is a privilege to review Dr. Bouchard's book, Live Longer And Stronger With Breast Cancer, an essential guide to support the most common cancer in women world wide with over 2 million new diagnosis per year. With so much information available at your fingertips today, it can be incredibly difficult to determine which path to take. Dr. Bouchard helps "underwhelm your overwhelm" by helping you navigate the cancer journey from the initial shock wave of diagnosis, overcoming the "why me" phase, and offering tangible and powerful action steps in a simple to follow, well rounded, with focus on the individual beyond the tumor, to produce the very best outcomes. Her words are a much needed light illuminating your path back to wellness."

- Dr. Nasha Winters, ND, FABNO

Dedication

To all the past, current and future patients of Inside Health Clinic, the warriors and inspirational heroes who I have had the pleasure to help. Thanks for putting your trust in me with your health journey.

Table of Contents

• CHAPTER 1 •

The Common Reaction, "Me? Cancer? What?!"

Never in a million years would you think you would be told, "You have cancer". The breast cancer diagnosis is terrifying – it's a diagnosis you hoped you'd never hear. You feel too young to have to deal with the symptoms, upcoming appointments, stress, side effects of drugs, extreme low energy, insomnia, pain, and not to mention the mental stress and how it will impact your family and loved ones. You love your life, and going over this hurdle was never a part of the plan. Living a long and healthy life is the only plan.

BUT, CANCER DOESN'T RUN IN MY FAMILY.

Did the diagnosis totally shock you? Yes. Does breast cancer even run in your family? Nope. Up until the diagnosis you were "healthy" and had never suspected cancer to be in your near future. You have done everything in your life right. You have listened to your general practitioner and did as they suggested. You attended your yearly checkups, never missed a single appointment, and here you are. Are you still feeling like you are missing information? Missing a reason? Are you asking yourself daily, what now? Are you wondering if there is something else out there but you have not yet grasped it?

Have you found yourself questioning the medical process? Are you getting the best possible care during this time? What about your treatment – how can you help your body heal? Asking questions and being unsure of this journey is okay. There is more and you do have options.

Google searches and various anti-cancer books start to become overwhelming. Which diet is best for you? Should you get your hormones checked? What are the best ways to boost your immune system and to live longer? There is a lot of information out there and you need to know what is best for you, your body, and your cancer. You are indeed different than every other cancer patient, and therefore you need specific and individualized care.

After each chemo session, you will feel your

body become weaker and weaker. You will know the chemo drugs are wreaking havoc on your system. It is something you will see, smell, and feel. Deep down, you know that chemo and drugs can not be your only option. You want your body and immune system to get stronger, because you have a better chance at fighting this disease if your immune system is on your side.

You're ready to take back the power; instead of waiting for a miracle you want to take control of your own life. Without taking this step towards having ownership of your health you will worry and have anxiety about your future. You will always be waiting for that next appointment; flipping a coin or playing Russian roulette. There is obviously something that has gone wrong that has led you down this path, and now you realize, better late than never, that it would be crazy to keep doing the same thing while expecting a different result.

Maybe being optimistic has always been a part of who you are. Do you feel lucky to have supportive loved ones around you, reminding you to keep pushing forward, and trusting in yourself and the journey? Do you feel love and gratefulness to be alive and are you determined to stop this disease from taking over your life, physically and mentally?

The more you learn about health, you will realize, "Okay, maybe my lifestyle hasn't been perfect, but whose is?" The diagnosis has made you want to do something, make changes to be healthier, so you can live stronger and longer with your family. It is up to you to take the power and responsibility for your health back, and I will help show you how.

IT DOESN'T MAKE SENSE

It doesn't make any logical sense that you have been diagnosed with cancer. There is no history of any cancer in your family, and doctors have always said that you are healthy and doing great at all of your yearly physicals. You don't do drugs, and would only drink a few glasses of wine socially to relax or celebrate an occasion. You only take Advil or Tylenol once in a while when you have cramps or have a migraine. Your energy has always been on the low to moderate side, and yes, you're likely holding onto some extra weight, but that's the extent of your "complaints".

As far as diet, you have been a part of various weight loss programs for years; you're a huge fan of following schedules and routines. You liked these programs: the easy to prepare meals which are portioned properly. Going out to eat and ordering in probably happens more often than you'd like to admit, but when life is crazy busy you just want something fast and convenient. You always chose the healthier options anyways: The pita place with nitrate and MSG filled toppings can't be that bad, right? When in a rush, pasta with a meat sauce is always a staple in your house, because it is fast and easy to make and besides, it provides the nutrition of the four food groups, right? You may also have a sweet tooth, but who doesn't? Especially before you menstrate or when you're stressed. Those are credible reasons for sugar cravings. Maybe you skip breakfast and then maybe also lunch. Your life is hectic and coffee usually keeps you fuelled throughout the day. On a daily basis you could potentially be drinking up to four to six cups of coffee without ever really noticing. Tons of people eat way worse than you do and have more stress and chaotic lives than you do, and they don't have cancer. So why you?

THE FIGHTING SPIRIT

The question, "Why you?" Is unfortunately not something we can pin down and provide a reason for through an internet search. But what I can tell you is this: You are a fighter. Throughout diagnosis, treatment, appointments, continuing to wake up each day, remaining positive while feeling your worst, you have proven that you are willing to do anything it takes to overcome this disease.

After chemo, you realize the chances of your cancer spreading or coming back is much higher in the first two to five years, and that there is so much more that you can do to keep your body strong in the meantime. Doctors may not always have all the answers and together you both need to start searching outside the box. You've often Googled: "best therapies for cancer", or "how to beat cancer", or "reverse this disease", and often only the medical jargon and pharmaceutical drugs pop up as the one and only option. These results not only make you feel like shit, they are shit.

You need to understand firstly **why** you have cancer, and secondly **what** you can do to feel better NOW and **how** you can start supporting your body to fight cancer better. Knowing everything you can about your cancer and how you can strengthen your body will increase your chances of survival. Having an integrative and comprehensive plan to fight cancer will be your new life force.

Your cancer will be one of, if not the only, ultimate battle that you will encounter in your lifetime. Sure, you will have your ups and downs, frustrations, sadness, and moments of fear and uncertainty, but overall, nothing can stand in your way to keep strong and keep plowing through the obstacles that you will face. You will say, *"F*ck cancer"*. You will do anything to live longer, have more energy, and gain more quality time with your family throughout this process because you have a fighting spirit.

My dream is to give you the guidance and tools to live longer in the face of cancer, as I know the human spirit is full of possibilities and I can help guide you to making this your reality.

• CHAPTER 2 •

Doctor: A Researcher and Investigator

IT'S IN MY BLOOD

Since birth, I have lived in a world bombarded by sesame hemp balls and extensive poop talk. I was raised in a home where the benefits of natural medicine were preached daily by my age-defying mother. My mother is extremely passionate and well educated in the field of health sciences as well as holistic methods. By profession, she is a registered nurse and has spent many years helping women in delivery rooms and she has also been educated by Dr. Bernard Jenson, who is one of the forefathers of natural healing and he has reversed many chronic diseases by focusing on gut health.

My brother, sister and I rarely had visits to the doctor's office since we were rarely sick. My mom had everything our immune systems needed as well as important remedies tucked away in every cabinet, drawer, and nook in our kitchen. I remember having breakfast in the mornings as a child and I would wonder if my friends would also be seated to a feast of fresh food alongside a handful of supplements supplied by their mothers like I was?

I definitely felt like a *weirdo* while attending grade school. *'Weirdo'* is the best word to describe how I felt about myself and truly how my peers made me feel about the daily routines in my household. My friends would scrunch their noses and furrow their brows at my homemade lunches and laugh at the idea that my mother would place dandelion sprouts in my tuna sandwiches. Thinking about it presently, it makes me laugh because I have a clear memory of myself examining my daily lunch and thinking similarly to my friends expressions, "What the F%*K is in my lunch now?" My mom would also try to be super sneaky, like adding pine seeds and chlorophyll to any snack possible. But in the end, I never had an ear infection, or skin issue, and always had a ton of energy. So deep down in my heart, I knew that my mother knew her shit, metaphorically as well as literally and when reflecting back on my childhood, it is not surprising that I chose to study naturopathic medicine.

Oddly enough, as a child, I always thought going to the doctors and getting medicine/ antibiotics or checked out by an expert was a "privilege". I would often wonder, "Why can't I go on antibiotics?" and I was always envious of my friends who did. It's a strange concept, but I think I may have equated doctor visits and appointments to important and quality time with my mom, or maybe I just liked the idea and attention of being checked up on by someone who was not my mom. Either way, I was always excited to see the doctor and felt it was a requirement of having a normal childhood.

My mother would tell me, "Your body can heal itself when given the right tools". She has the medical background to know when things are beyond our bodies self healing abilities, and knew when a trip to the emergency room was needed, but thankfully that was never an occurrence growing up in my family home. My mother always had a clear understanding that our body is made up of a mixture of chemical reactions, vitamins, and minerals and when those are thrown off balance, symptoms occur. We are just one big self-healing mechanism that when provided all of the necessary tools, our bodies will get back into a harmonious balance and start to reverse disease. It is a unique chemistry that makes up all of our bodies and seems miraculous that our bodies can self heal and seek balance when provided the right tools.

TRUST YOUR GUT: IT'S A SUPER POWER

Why are moms always right? It's annoying isn't it? Even as an adult, I still feel like my mother can read a room and her assumptions become reality. A mother's intuition is actually incredible. When I would seek advice, she would respond and say to me, "What does your gut say?", "Trust your gut", or "Follow your gut feeling". I feel blessed to humbly say, I have learned to trust my gut and intuition because of my mother's teachings and feel confident that it could never lead me astray. She always preached the importance of us focusing on the gut (for decision making, as well as for overall health), and it took me four years of post-graduate work and a year into clinical practice to really believe the true depth of the gut as a healing power.

"The journey of health begins in the gut."

Another popular topic at our dinner table when I was growing up was poop. It wasn't strange for mom to ask: "What does it look like?", "Pieces of food in it?", "Does it sink or float?", "Let me have a look! I want to see the size and shape!". To think that the topic of 'poop' is only now becoming popular within medical communities and only now is gaining more scientific publicity is amazing since it has been a part of my daily discussions my whole life. Terms like; "microbiome", "gut health", or "gut is our second brain" are now a part of medical communities everyday lingo and from an expert's point of view, I would arguably say that the gut is our first brain.

After Naturopathic medical school, my head was packed with so much information. Four years of learning intensely about the human body, how it works, what to do to keep everything in balance, and I still thought the idea of the body being self healing could not be that simple. Could it?!

I'll never forget my first, most complicated patient, G.L., who came to me right when I was fresh out of school. G.L. had seen neurologists, ear/nose/and throat specialists, and conventional doctors regarding his fatigue and debilitating migraines. Being placed on several medications with no success, he decided to try a more natural route. It was only after thorough gut cleaning and the rebuilding of his adrenals and nervous system that he was able to get back to work, and regain his life. More medication was not the answer. It took time and patience, but even now, 10 years later he is enjoying his wonderful activity filled life and feeling happy and healthy doing it.

Figuring out health issues from the gut on a cellular level has always made the most sense to me. It is the 21st Century and I think it is time for people to begin to truly heal mentally and physically and realize that the outdated "band-aid" approach is suppressing and not working. Today – these holistic and natural concepts or 'weird things' are now our fastest growing industry. A large portion of our population is trying 'Plant Based' lifestyles. Juicing celery and inventing the next best keto snack are two of the many new innovations created daily. I am excited that these "trends" are making noise. Millions of people around the world are becoming more in tune with their own bodies and learning ways to provide it proper nutrition which is needed to be stronger, last longer, and heal faster.

THINKING OUTSIDE THE BOX

By the time I turned 18 years old, I knew my life was going in a direction outside the traditional "mainstream" healing. At the time, this thought of gut health was so far from the norm that I had to learn more and I had to really research and dive my nose into books to find answers.

Why was I rarely sick? Why did others have their tonsils or appendix removed? And why don't I ever suffer, like my friends, with infections? This is the frame of mind that led me to want to become a Naturopathic Doctor and understand the complexities of the body, and how to prevent disease on a physiological and biological level. To me, this always made sense as true health care.

When starting my practice, my first patients were chronically ill, and I knew more water and the correct nutrition was not everything; they would need much more. What else could a Naturopathic Doctor do to heal the people who have, without knowing it, been unwell most of their lives, and are now labelled with a "disease?" Most of the time, we are raised with poor lifestyle choices, such as fast foods that are over-processed and contain too much sugar. In busy households, it's likely habitual to eat take-out, or pre-made foods that are microwaved and deep-fried. Food items prepared in this way eliminate all nutritional value, but the convenience of these options in the 80's, 90's, and 2000's was irresistibly tempting. We didn't know that there was anything wrong with being raised this way, so people continued to teach these lifestyle habits to their children without ever realizing the consequences.

It is nice to know that we are now living in a world where we are becoming more aware of health choices and continuing this education is key. Taking preventative measures is the best way to live a healthy life. By educating yourself and knowing what is harmful to your body and then staying far away from it is the absolute best practice to staying healthy. But... when you are diagnosed with cancer – a diagnosis that likely blew your mind – it opens up a whole world of questions, such as, *"Why me?"*

Let me tell you something that may resonate: Every person and their own cancer experience is going to be different from yours. Breast cancer specifically takes years to grow in the body, so by the time you found your lump, it was likely five to ten years in the making. The most successful cancer patients that I have worked with are willing to change their entire life. You need to start thinking positively and change the question of, *"Why me?"* to the question, **"What now?"** Try to see cancer as a blessing and be willing to make big changes in your life. You will feel healthier than you've ever felt by feeding your body the way it's meant to be fed. You will realize your body's incredible self healing abilities, and negate many of the habits that speed cancers growth.

Treating cancer is the ultimate challenge. The process of peeling away the layers of what makes cancer grow is exciting – Was it your ongoing stress? Was it being mentally and emotionally overwhelmed? Was it the job you didn't like? Was it the garbage food you put in your body all these years without knowing it? What about your mother's health, and her mother's health?

We are all a by-product of what came before us. Was your mother a smoker or around secondhand smoke? The answers to these questions are what doctors need to know in order to get your whole body clean to fight the ultimate battle.

TREATING *YOU*, NOT JUST THE CANCER

I do not see cancer as an intimidating fight; the strongest survivors I work with are the ones who know they are up for any challenge and have faith that the cancer wasn't going to take over their lives. Whether you just recently finished chemotherapy and radiation, had a recent surgery, or did not take that path at all, the goal here is to boost your immune system and keep you strong to battle anything that comes your way.

Even after patients come to me with only "a few months left to live," I never let this prognosis intimidate my practice. Practitioners and clinicians know that patients who are doing all the things that are proven to prolong life – using strategies that will make them feel stronger and healthier, are not just another statistic. In the search for all the top cancer-fighting tools, I travelled all over the world to understand what the world's stance on cancer was. I also sought out answers for how to survive and fight against it. And surprisingly, survival comes down to a simple strategy: 1) the strength of an individual (emotionally and physically) and 2) the knowledge and equipment one carries in order to charge into this battle. That is the ultimate goal – feeling your best, with confidence that the cancer doesn't stand a chance in coming back. When you live with this awareness, you can be a better person, parent, become more present with your family, be more in tune at your job, and point your energy in the right direction, living life with purpose. Cancer does not own your future. You are an incredible healer, and when given the right tools and knowledge, you become unstoppable.

It's your strength and determination to survive that empowers me to become a better Doctor, constantly researching new ways to keep your body strong. I put myself in your shoes, and understand you want to do everything in your power to not only survive, but to also thrive in the face of cancer. Your strength, passion for your family, and determination to survive is the reason why you're reading this book – to learn everything you can to fight cancer more effectively and live longer.

MY CLINICAL FOCUS

Deep down in my core, I've always loved seeing others happy. Seeing someone ill and helpless breaks my heart, which is why I gravitated to the health field in the first place. All throughout Naturopathic Medical School, everything just clicked; when it came to the human body, I just loved learning everything about it. Naturopathic Medical School is a four year post graduation program that is similar to conventional medical school, however instead of the prime focus being pharmaceutical drugs, there is a large focus on herbal medicine, acupuncture, homeopathy, clinical nutrition, and hydrotherapy. In my last year of medical school, my peers and I got to apply for clinical specialty shifts and the thought of focusing on oncology frightened me. I assumed that oncology was a depressing field in general, so I felt for me (being a naturally super optimistic positive human being) that applying for this shift would be a big mistake, so I didn't. Instead, I applied for the mental health shift...You read correctly!...How ironic! Right? Each week I helped people with anxiety, schizophrenia, OCD, and depression; but because of this experience I have so much more insight on how mental health affects your body physically and why being positive in the most difficult circumstances can be helpful when rejuvenating your body's strength.

Shortly after I graduated, I opened up my own naturopathic clinic, called Inside Health. My clinic includes services to assist and optimize the body's own healing ability, such as nutrition through intravenous therapy, colon hydrotherapy, stress management, and a large emphasis on whole body healing and nutrition. Opening Inside Health was an extremely exciting time. I was a naïve 24 year old, passionate about healing, and was given the opportunity to offer a variety of health services to **ANYONE** who wanted the help. It was my ultimate dream come true.

People often ask me, "Why chose to focus your practice on cancer?"   My inspiration really originates with my patients and what I have learned from them and how I have been able to help them.

My first cancer patient (let's call him D.Y.) came into my clinic and was literally slumped over in his chair. He physically was unable to hold his own weight, he sat supported by his incredible wife, saying he had been told he was in his last few months, but was not ready to die. He was no longer responding to any chemotherapy treatments; there was nothing left for him in the mainstream world of medicine. I thought, "Why is the universe putting him in my office after a one-month palliative diagnosis was given? What can I provide that the mainstream hasn't?"

Well, here's the truth – that man changed how I thought about cancer. D.Y.'s determination to survive and see the birth of his second grandchild kept his mind focused and driven to survive. There was no holding him back. He listened to every protocol and every remedy that I recommended. His body was knocked down to such a degree, that every organ was suffering. The combination of injections, nutrition, colon hydrotherapy, heavy metal chelation and detoxification was what turned his body around. This intense protocol along with his powerful mindset was exactly what his body needed to create miracles.

Even years later, his oncologist wondered, "How are you still alive?"

Over the years, my passion for understanding cancer grew. I travelled all over the United States, Canada, and even Germany, to understand what the leaders in oncology were doing. I was always on top of the research, protocols, and best practice, as they are always changing, but the underlying function of what makes a body healthy has been known for hundreds of years. When it comes to cancer – I have always put myself in my patients shoes – I think, "What would I do if I had this diagnosis? What if that was my mother or father? What kind of protocol would I create to keep them alive longer?" I strive to discover every possibility and never leave any stone unturned.

After eight years of remission, post-palliative diagnosis, I am so grateful for having the opportunity to meet D.Y. and all the other cancer thrivers I've helped throughout the years. My patients have taught me the true strength and determination a single person can have. I no longer fear treating cancer because now I have learned how to fight it more effectively.

I put my heart and soul into every person who walks into the clinic and who truly wants to get well. I want you to have the best results. Knowing you are unique and have a special story, I want to work with you to make sure you do everything you can to live a longer and stronger life.

Within the first year of clinical practice, I knew right away that my approach to cancer would be different, and I would use tools beyond what conventional medicine and any other naturopathic clinic had to offer.

THE MIRACLES

I have studied with integrative doctors, whose main focus was not just to help people feel better, but to actually reverse disease within their patients. The miracles I have seen are mind-blowing, and I knew I had to constantly expand my learning and update my research on what works – that is the only way my patients will get long-term positive health. Health is not "one size fits all." Every person is unique and has a special story. This individuality is what makes the health profession so interesting, and not one person with cancer will ever present cancer symptoms in the same way.

I have been lucky to meet several patients who turned to me when they were at death's door. When they had no other choices or options from the conventional field, they turned to me – "Ah hem, so I'm your last resort?!"... I am actually thrilled by this! Believe it or not, those are my favorite types of patients – the ones who are willing to do everything possible to survive because there is nothing else. These patients are willing to adjust their life, because they know that how they've been living has led them here. It's never too late to turn your health around and the people who seek my help are so willing that it brings tears to my eyes. I love the passion and will to survive; there's a special power to the ones who never quit. I love helping the people who want to do everything it takes in order to live a longer and stronger life despite their diagnosis or prognosis.

THE APPROACH TAKEN OF A REBEL

From a young age, for some reason, I've always enjoyed doing the opposite of what others told me to do. I love proving others wrong. It is a trait that my friends and family would sometimes term: annoying, but it is my most proud quality. It is this exact behavior that gives me tremendous joy in seeing someone extend their life against all odds. Even when patients are told that they only have a "month to live", I know collectively we can do everything in our power to ensure that this is not true. No one can put a number on your life, until you've done everything it takes to live longer, and I absolutely love proving those statistics wrong.

My passion lies in getting people out of the way of death's doorstep and helping turn their lives around. When given the right tools, your body has the ability to reverse disease, even cancer.

Being a Naturopathic Doctor, my approach is different from chemotherapy, radiation, and all the medications that are offered by conventional medicine. These conventional therapies can only get your body so far. After listening to your story, reviewing your lab work, ordering additional "outside of mainstream" tests, and after a thorough physical exam is performed, I put a plan into place. We do not want to accept the cancer statistics and will do everything in to help you fight with all the means available to strengthen your body.

Your body is intuitive and powerful; when you remove all the obstacles and barriers and feed it proper nutrition, it has the ability to become stronger and fight abnormal cells, including cancer. I chose to focus on breast cancer in this book because it strikes me in the very heart of the matter, being a woman, a mother to my children, and a spouse to my husband. A diagnosis can happen at any age, but more commonly I see women who are within their child bearing years and this makes them more relatable to where I am in my life. I often find myself thinking, what protocol would I put myself on, knowing how hungry I am for life. All these women have such a strong will to thrive, children to raise, businesses and partners they love, and an overall passion for life. You fighting cancer is about doing everything you can to find balance in the body, giving it love, and investigating why the balance is off kilter in the first place.

Looking at the body as a whole, not just the cancer, is the key to getting well, and this means supporting your immune system, gut health, nervous system, stress glands, emotional health, and healing past traumas. Healing on all levels fights cancer more effectively and will allow you to live a longer and healthier life. I want to guide you through all the steps that are needed to live longer, despite your diagnosis, and I want you to feel empowered by your cancer, learning all there is to know about your body along the way.

• CHAPTER 3 •

Needed to Fight Breast Cancer

This book is a step-by-step guide, giving you all the tools needed to understand and fight your cancer more effectively. Each step will provide homework, checklists, and resources to ensure that you are ready to move forward and prolong your life.

The first thing that I would recommend you do is to remember that the key to organizing and understanding the massive amounts of information you will begin to immediately receive is "underwhelm the overwhelm". With the overwhelming amount of information you receive from friends, loved ones, professional opinions, and even Dr. Google, it is easy to get confused about where to start and what is best for your body. (Remember that cancer is not a "one size fits all" disease.) This guide will help you understand that, before you even jump into treatment options and the steps included in this book, you need the right mindset to drive your success. This is an exciting time; checking in on how you view your cancer, understanding your purpose, and giving yourself the compassion you need is important to fight this disease effectively. It's time to find your tribe, the people, and support group that will motivate you to keep looking forward and motivating your health and longevity.

THE STEPS

Knowing your body

Our body is complex, and in order to understand how to live longer, we must understand how our body functions. We are striving for ultimate health. So knowing the basic functions of our digestive and nervous system, our stress response, and how our detox organs perform day-to-day is crucial information to understand when implementing immediate strategies to help our own body function better.

Answering Questions

The next step is to understand answers to these questions: 'What is breast cancer?', 'What are the different types?', 'How did I get it?', and 'What stimulates its growth?' and throughout learning the answers to these questions, you will certainly come across cancer jargon that you have never seen before. Learning cancer terminology is important in order to fight cancer in a powerful way.

Food and Nutrition

Another huge part of fighting cancer effectively is knowing which foods we should, or should not, put into our body. Food is such an important topic, and you will learn all the foods that directly enhance immune function, as well as the ones that set your body back and have been directly linked to stimulating cancerous growth. When it comes to diet, the next step is to learn strategies and rules around eating. For example: you will learn how restricting the times you eat can play a powerful role in fighting your cancer. You will also learn how, when, and what to eat, according to your breast cancer.

Included in this book is a two-week plan on how to eat; prepping your body for the next step in your fight against cancer. For weekly and monthly meal plans you can refer to the back of the book at any time for an easy-to-access reference guide on what meals to add to your life based on where you are in the process.

Detoxification

Once you have all the foundational information, we need to take things to the next level – detoxification. We want to clear your body of all the garbage that is clinging to your insides; anything that is holding your body back from fighting cancer day-to-day needs to go. Optimizing how your body functions to clear and detoxify is something you can apply in your daily life; however, in that section of the book, you will also learn the step-by-step process of how to detox your body on the deepest level: for optimal energy, immunity, lymphatic, digestive, and nervous system health. This is the secret weapon to living longer with breast cancer, and I have included a seven-day detoxification accelerator program, designed to keep you accountable and on track for healing.

Data and Testing

After the detoxification process, you will take time to get quantifiable data determining where you are in your cancer battle. You will learn which tests are involved, which ones are a waste of time, and which ones can help you understand what is going on in your body on a cellular level so you can create a personalized plan for moving forward. These tests will determine what other obstacles are standing in your way toward health. These tests set a baseline of where you are, and what else needs to be done. This brings us to the last step – the cancer-specific treatments needed to live longer. In this chapter, you will learn which treatments have the most research for treating breast cancer. These individualized therapies and protocols are explained in order to accelerate your cancer-killing results.

Perspective and Enlightenment

You are about to emerge into a whole new world of healing and learning, and your perspective on how to treat any disease (especially your breast cancer) will become a process that you are in control of. Incredible things will start to happen and I am so excited for you to embrace this journey. Giving yourself time and space to really dig deep to understand yourself will always give you the best results. You are worthy of healing and success – so get ready to start your new chapter!

STEP 1: Thinking like a Cancer Survivor

When fighting cancer effectively you must have the right mindset. You have always been a fighter and have always done what it takes to get through tough times; this fight is no different. When you think like a survivor, you will be one. This will likely be the most important fight of your life, and there are key traits you can learn in order to not only fight cancer cells more effectively, but to also live stronger and longer.

MINDSET

It has been scientifically proven that when you are optimistic, minimize stress and have a strong will to survive, your chances of survival after cancer occurrence will be increased. This is demonstrated through a study with breast cancer patients who received psychological interventions to support their mindset and psychology; they proved to have a 45 percent reduced risk of breast cancer recurrence, and 59 percent reduced risk of death from breast cancer.[1] Asking for help is key, since being optimistic is not always easy, and yes, you will have bad days – that's within human nature – but overall, it's your passion for life and living with purpose that will make this journey successful.

When fear sets in, it's merely a survival mechanism. When you start wondering about all the "what ifs?" and "what does the future hold?" and you start questioning every decision, you will soon realize that this mentality gets you nowhere! Fear makes us feel as if we have limited options and keeps us stagnant. When we start thinking about how we can do things differently and what steps need to be taken to move forward, we start to see results. The fastest way to get rid of fear is to *take action*.

TAKE ACTION

Having a cancer diagnosis forces you out of your comfort zone and demands that you take action. Realizing that you have so much more control and choices for your body than what the conventional health model has to offer, and trying an integrative approach will help decrease this fear of the unknown or fear of not having any control. Trying new things, discovering what makes you feel your best, and seeing results, will help to dissipate this fear.

But still, *what if it doesn't work?* Luckily you are fortunate to have access to objective data to see what stage your cancer has progressed to: MRIs, ultrasounds, imaging, labs and testing to monitor where you are with your cancer, and this data will help you assess whether your current plan is effective. With active cancer, I recommend evaluating every 1-3 months to see blood markers change and tumor size shrinking. If not, a more aggressive plan of action needs to happen. In general, even if the treatment plan is successful, cancer is smart, and there needs to be constant variation in your life purposely planned to outsmart these abnormal cancer cells. Listening to and knowing your body is a key strategy when fighting cancer. If you keep learning and adapting to change, you will eventually get to where you want to be – alive longer.

It's important to take the time to reflect, dig deep, and find your purpose and passion for being alive. What gives you that "get up and go" energy? That excitement that makes you not just want to be alive, but *feel* alive? Is it dancing or singing to your favorite song? Does your work, hobbies, or children fill you with this joy? What is it that gets you out of bed and motivates you to keep going? The journey of being diagnosed with breast cancer will change you and you will become a whole new person in the process. Throughout this journey, you may even find that your social network of friends, family and colleagues may change.

YOU ARE WHO YOU SURROUND YOURSELF WITH

You may have had this realization prior to your breast cancer diagnosis, and already made some changes. It is especially important that throughout this time you need a non-judgmental support group. So surround yourself with people who have the same mindset and who are optimistic, accepting, and love you. Surrounding yourself with people who do not support you will likely bring on frustration and anger. This is a transitional time in your life, and it is greatly encouraged to think about yourself without feeling guilty. Put strong boundaries around spending time with people who lift you up and make you feel strong.

Being around negative people is one of the most toxic things someone with cancer can do.

Having the power within yourself to address past feelings of anger, guilt, resentment, and to clear any misunderstandings in order to lighten any heaviness that your body is holding onto, is worth every ounce of positive energy it will provide to your health. Cancer can be a pivotal time in your life, and you need to think about yourself and be selfish. Find a group of people who will support you positively and remind you of why it's important to continue this fight on a daily basis. Reaching out to these people will help put your feelings into context. You are not alone in this journey and you are not a burden. If you google "cancer support" in your community area you will be pleasantly surprised that support groups do exist with women just like you. Finding your team of supporters will reaffirm how connected you are, and these social networks are an invaluable part of your healing process.[2] This sense of community is a big part of how Inside Health Clinic contributes to your healing. We ensure that you are surrounded with other like minded individuals, and you also receive encouragement and therapy without a formal therapy appointment.

Secondly, make sure to recognize and offload your stressors. What are the things that make your body feel drained and overwhelmed? Every time we perform a stressful act, or push our body to its limits, our adrenal glands release a hormone called cortisol. Most women, even prior to their diagnosis, have been functioning on high cortisol for years, which is why we can multi-task and accomplish so much in a single day. Heightened stress levels and higher cortisol are directly correlated with a weakened immune response. Having a diagnosis of cancer automatically puts you in the fight or flight response, so it is time to review your surroundings, and start getting comfortable asking for help, because if you don't, you will burn out.

After years of fulfilling the mom role within the family; Karen, who has Breast Cancer, realized if she continues with the "do it all" mindset and the stress that naturally comes with it, she will burn out and not be any use to her family at all. She was lucky enough to hire a "mother's helper" whose role was to come for three hours a day to help with groceries, tidying the house, and preparing dinner. If that is not financially possible for you, you can ask a friend to pick up groceries for you, or delegate other roles to people who will be more than happy to help. Asking for help and assistance with daily tasks is necessary for you to balance your hormones. We all need help at some point, so you need to ask.

BE SELFISH! FOR ONCE, PLEASE!

Over the years of treating cancer, I have seen a common trend where patients think of everyone else's needs first and put themselves last. They are always on the go, caring for their loved ones, and feel depleted at the end of each day. Thinking about yourself is likely a strange concept; especially when you're so used to spreading yourself so thin, caring for others. Taking time for yourself and for your healing may feel selfish. You most likely work too many hours and have a busy schedule. Taking time for yourself may even feel unproductive when you have a long list of things to do. This is the exact mindset that needs to be changed. Listening carefully to your body is key and reacting to its messages is something you will need to do.

Instead of creating these endless to-do lists and ignoring the signals that tell you to stop and slow down, I want you to literally shorten these endless to-do lists by at least a quarter. That's right, stop being an overachiever! Functioning because of passion creates a much different energy than doing things because of self pressure and judgement. If a friend or relative asks you to do something, and the thought of it doesn't lighten you, you must say no. Let me repeat that. It is okay to say no! Start a hot bath or pick up a book or start a new series on Netflix instead. Start making it a habit to only involve yourself with things that build your energy, versus stripping it away to benefit others.

COMPASSION FOR YOURSELF

In addition to being selfish for once, treat yourself the way you would want to treat an ill friend. Listen without judgement and rephrase your thoughts and comments. This is an important lesson in learning to stop judging yourself. For example, if you catch yourself saying, "I'm so stupid; why did I smoke cigarettes for so long," try turning it around and releasing that judgement. Instead, you can say, "It's okay, it's now time to make a change and look forward." When you treat yourself with acceptance, you do not exaggerate your mistakes into a negative misrepresentation of yourself. It's quite normal for these feelings to surface, so embrace them without criticism and judgment.

When A.K. first came into the clinic, she knew her cancer was the result of a perfect storm. She had worked long hours, she swallowed a decade of birth control pills, and had many emotional stressors causing her too many sleepless nights. Breast cancer surprisingly was not a shock to her. Something had to change. Incorporating a minimum of ten minutes a day of silence or guided meditation is an excellent way to give back to your body. Implementing mindful practices is a way A.K. took back her mind and soul in the face of a busy, crazy lifestyle.

Take a break from your to-do list. This can be done by sitting alone in a room and focusing on your breath, or by turning on the audio for a guided meditation, or taking an Epsom salt bath and allowing your body to relax and breathe. In addition, you can take yoga classes – either solo or in a group which guides your breathing as well as gets your blood moving. Practice anything that nurtures yourself and causes you to turn inwards to your body and breath. Most people who find yoga and meditation a challenge are the ones who need it the most; just like A.K., these are the kind of people whose minds are on everything except themselves, and they can't seem to direct their focus. This is the exact practice that will help strengthen your mind and body and keep your forward focus, rather than being distracted by everything and everyone around you. For A.K., this simple ten minute practice in the morning and at night allowed her to relax her mind, allowed her to get a deeper night's rest, resulting in feeling recharged the next day.

If a thought enters your mind, such as, "I cannot meditate," or, "Yoga is just not for me," then go back to the same notion of treating yourself like a friend. Would you ever tell a friend that something is just not for them? Despite it being researched as highly productive for their health? Or would you be that supportive person saying, "Yes, give it a try. What do you have to lose?" and having an open mind set and understanding that any new practice in your life will literally challenge you and will take practice to improve? Always give yourself the benefit of the doubt when trying new things, without judgement of perceived failure.

IT'S TIME TO GROW

Taking the time to learn about yourself and your reactions to this cancer journey will allow you to recognize growth and development in tough situations. Treat yourself with kindness and compassion, instead of self-blame or by punishing yourself through negative thought patterns. The section below is a short list of eight suggested homework tools to help turn around negative mindsets, and grow your positivity even when you feel that there is nothing left. For each point, I will give you guidance on how you can successfully implement these strategies into each and every day. Anyone at any time can do this homework to help promote a positive mindset. If you want to get your kids/partner/friends involved, please do!

Homework

1. When you wake up in the morning, before checking your phone, or thinking about your day, I want you to have a pen and paper within reach, and write a list of ten things that you are grateful for. These can be as simple as, "The sun is shining", " I have a roof over my head", or "I have a warm bed". Start your morning by showing gratitude for these simple things.

2. Celebrate any and all small accomplishments you have throughout your day. With cancer, things are constantly changing and evolving. Releasing endorphins and celebrating the small milestones will help keep your mind on the end goal – living longer. So what if these accomplishments are remembering to pick up your kids from school, or having a shower when you really didn't feel like it!

3. Start a journal and record the emotions you have during the day, what you did, and your

dreams and your goals. Writing down your sad moments, frustrations, and possible anger will act as a release, and you may be surprised at what comes out.

4. Remember to catch yourself with negative self-talk and release the judgements right away. In place of those initial feelings, immediately write down how you would like to feel instead. This journal will also help keep you focused regarding your dreams and goals for your future.

5. Reach out to loved ones and show them you care. You may be surprised how taking the time to reconnect with the ones who have impacted you has positive effects on your mood. On a more molecular level, there is a signaling protein found on all immune cells called CD4. Studies show that resentments, guilt and anger result in lower CD4 levels, equating to a weaker immune state.[3] In the long run, taking the time to heal resentments, anger, guilt will have a powerful effect on your immune system; therefore, your immune fighting cells can increase and focus

on their number one job, to fight cancer cells.

6. Create time to escape reality. Pick up a lighthearted fictional book. Taking your mind off the stressors of your life and digging into another world will act as a mental break. With all the research you do and serious conversations you have, now is the time to take a break and allow yourself to look at life through another person's eyes. Aim for one exciting new fictional book each month, if that sounds stressful, make it every 2-3 months tops. If you are not a book lover, escape reality by getting together with friends at least once a week and have this be "cancer free" conversation.

7. Unplug from the internet. Start with every evening, shutting off your phone and laptop from 6pm onwards. Next, only allow yourself to be on social media or run free with internet searches for a maximum of 2 hours each day. The internet can be an overwhelming world, and it is easy to wrap yourself up in social media platforms such as Facebook, and Instagram etc. You may even feel disheartened by comparing

yourself to others. Do yourself a huge favor by limiting all the visual stimulants that are distracting your mind and taking energy away from your healing.

8. Find something to laugh about every day. Laughter can be your best medicine. Putting on a comedy channel on television, laughing at yourself, or any other forms of humor can help you take the edge off and not take life as seriously. On a physiological level, laughter significantly improves your immune system's natural killer cells fighting activity within 12 hours of watching humorous videos.4 After all, that's what life is all about – enjoying the moments we have.

9. Make sleep a priority! Sleeping has a drastic effect on how you regulate mood and how you handle tough situations. Going to bed early, getting a comfortable pillow and bedding, and making your room completely dark can make a world of difference. Even if your days are long, and you feel that an extra hour of being awake will be exciting and needed, and you are feeling

an overwhelming sense of F.O.M.O. (aka the fear of missing out). I want you to try to forget about all of that. You need to discover how you feel when heading to bed at least an hour earlier.

For maximum energy and well being, your homework is to practice getting to sleep by 10:00pm and waking by 6:00am.

As you complete the homework, you may find that you already do these daily practices. If you do not, it's okay to start by taking baby steps and incorporating them slowly into your life. Each one will help optimize your mindset during your cancer healing journey. It is now time to think about yourself as a cancer survivor, not as a cancer patient. This is your time to take action, battle fear, re-examine your life, and take hold of this journey to transformation.

Step 2: Understanding the Body to keep it Healthy

"Natural forces within us are the true healers of disease." – Hippocrates

Most people know very little about how their body operates. We do not give our body much credit. Most of our knowledge about our body comes from learning about the basics at a very young age from health class or from our peers experiences, we are taught by what we see and read about in the media, and from our doctors recommendations, which is usually a drug to "cure" our health issues.

The belief that our body has the ability to heal itself when given the right nutrients is now seen as "alternative" medicine, when this kind of medicine should not be "alternative" at all, but should be considered a primary source. When treating a condition with a drug, you suppress what the body naturally tries to do on its own. For example, when your skin is scratched or cut, your innate intelligence knows the exact steps needed to heal your skin. When someone has cancer, there is something off balance in their body, and it is screaming for help to heal. We are not used to this mindset. Suppressing symptoms without knowing whether they are physical or mental is a large contributor to how we got sick in the first place. We need to look at our body as a whole and understand what causes it to go astray, what is deficient, what it is compensating for, and only then can we become strong enough to fight any disease that comes our way, especially cancer.

OUR LIFE VESSEL

We were all born with an amazing vessel that we call our body; it is continuously growing, evolving, healing, and changing. Every day, our heart beats for us and allows us to perform tasks without consciously telling it what to do. When it comes to survival, believe it or not, our body knows best. Imagine being in a stressful situation (this should be easy); your nervous system automatically tightens blood vessels in order to increase how fast your heart pumps blood throughout your body, your lungs expand to allow more air into your system, your pupils widen, so you can focus more clearly, and you have goose bumps, called piloerection, another survival mechanism used to make body hair stick out to increase how your body retains heat. Lastly, all blood flows directly away from your gut, slowing the function of your intestines. Our body naturally reacts this way in order to protect us from the stress we are enduring and naturally knows what to do. This is incredible.

Without realizing it, most of us are constantly living in a "fight or flight response." We live in a "go, go, go" type of world, where our body interprets everything as an emergency, with no time to rest. How can your body digest food properly when in this state? When you are in a state of anxiety, fear, or tension your body connects to its sympathetic nervous system which is also known as its survival mode. This is a good thing because if a bear is chasing you, this is how your body would help you stay alive. However, most situations we face are not emergencies, and learning how our body functions on a daily basis, and how it changes and shifts naturally in specific situations and circumstances is important so we can keep it healthy and avoid burning out.

STRESS RESPONSE

It is a fact that after any traumatic experience in your life (i..e. a cancer diagnosis), subconsciously, your body automatically goes into fear mode – fight or flight – or survival response. While waiting for an oncologist appointment or review imaging, your mind starts to think of every possible scenario, and with these thoughts your body will react. Your heart palpitations will get harder and faster; you begin to feel your temperature rising, your face flushes, you may begin to feel nauseous, and you may even start to perspire at just the thought of these situations.

The main organ that allows our body to deal with stress is called the adrenal glands. We have two of them and they are a large part of how our body deals with stress. They release cortisol to deal with the stress, and to help you carry on with life. When we have high cortisol, it not only slows down activity and energy to our digestive system, but it also suppresses our immune system and how it fights for us. Therefore, this is critical information to understand when it comes to maximizing how our bodies fight abnormal cells and kill cancer cells. We want to do everything in our power to support adrenal function and lessen this stress response, and yes, this can be trained.

Sleep

First off, it is important to receive a full night's rest; as mentioned previously, you should aim to be in bed by 10:00pm and awake by 6:00am. When your body is in a resting state your immune system works best and stress glands are able to rebuild and repair. If you are not sleeping for at least six solid hours per night doing so needs to be the first step to healing your body and keeping it strong. An important hormone called melatonin is only produced at night. When your melatonin level is low, it is linked to insomnia and depression. It's important to have your room pitch dark, since any light (including light from digital screens) will block our bodies ability to produce it. There are hundreds of other functions melatonin has, the main one being a powerful antioxidant.[1]

In a clinic, when testing levels of this hormone, it's interesting to see that almost all patients with cancer have low levels of melatonin, especially the ones who have worked shift work and who have been exposed to bright lights within a twenty four hour period. Can you see the vicious cycle? Low levels of melatonin further lead to a future restless nights sleep. In order to heal properly, it is imperative that we regulate circadian rhythms.

To improve your sleep, you must cut out all stimulants. Consider practicing meditation and breathing exercises, which are extremely effective anxiolytics, which means they decrease anxiety and help calm our nervous system to help relax. There has been wonderful clinical feedback on the use of weighted blankets -especially in cases of anxiety. The additional pressure appears to reduce the fight or flight arousal center in our nervous system, and encourage relaxation which will help you sleep more soundly throughout the night.

Supplements for Sleep

You can always talk to your health care provider about supplementing with other agents that balance sleep rhythm and calm your nervous system. Melatonin is my top choice for any shift worker or chronic insomniac who needs help setting a regular night time rhythm because of its additional anti-cancer benefits (described in the Advanced Treatment chapter). If the sleep issue is restless mind and anxiety the combination of passionflower, valerian root, GABA, tryptophan, and magnesium glycinate are recommended. Additionally, you can start a bedtime routine that incorporates herbal teas with chamomile, and/or peppermint or avena sativa. These herbal remedies all help calm your overactive brain to promote rest. There are many sleep combinations that would contain all of these, which tend to be very safe. Ask your doctor to see which recommendation they think is right for you.

Start each day with a release!

Waking up in the morning is the best time for your body to get rid of waste that the immune system has collected and shuttled to your colon throughout the night. That's right – you should have a large bowel movement in the morning. No matter what you've heard in the past, pooping must be done at least once a day, and depending on the volume of food you take in, you should poop approximately eighteen hours after every meal. The following is a checklist of how your poop should look and how you should feel:

- No pieces of food in it
- Fully formed
- Medium brown in color
- No mucous or slimy looking pieces attached
- No blood
- No sense of urgency or cramping prior to movement

We can tell a lot about our health based on what our poop looks like, and I encourage you to start a diary or add a section to your daily journal dedicated to poop to track what is processed and coming out of your body. If your bowel movements do not look like the statements above, you must keep reading to learn how to resolve these issues by optimizing your gut.

DIGESTION

Now, let's talk about food and what it takes for ultimate absorption of nutrients. Digestion begins as soon as you think about what you are going to eat or when you see your food. Our salivary glands start secreting enzymes (or, what my mother used to call "pac-men" as a child). These enzymes are located all along our digestive tract, starting in the mouth. These enzymes, and the action of chewing, are a critical step in our digestion. Generally, most of us would benefit from chewing more often and slower. There are many foods that need enzymes specifically from our mouth secreted from the process of chewing and without this process these foods would not be broken down at all in any other step within your digestive system – like corn.

When eating, you must be in what's called a "parasympathetic state," which is the opposite of the sympathetic state mentioned previously (i.e. survival mode). In order for all energy and attention to go to your gut in order to process your food entirely, you should avoid eating while driving, while doing errands, or while on a stressful phone call. Instead, you should eat when you are in a relaxed state and are one-hundred percent focused on chewing slowly and allowing your body time to absorb the nutrients being ingested. You want to aim for at least ten chews of each bite before you swallow. This may seem unnecessary when you compare this slower pace to the fast pace that the majority of the population eats their food, but with practice this will soon become your normal eating habit and the practice of wolfing down food on the run will become a distant memory.

Stomach Acid Testing

Once food enters your stomach, a powerful enzyme called hydrochloric acid is activated. Many of us have felt this acid when we experience heartburn, and as unpleasant of a feeling this is, the acid is important and allows our body to break down proteins into amino acids, which are the building blocks for our hormones and immune system. With age and stress, we produce less of this important stomach acid, resulting in gas and bloating. If you experience gas and bloat after a meal, I would suggest that you try the hydrochloric (HcL) test. You can start with taking 250mg of hydrochloric acid in supplement form with your next meal. If you get any type of pressure in your chest or heartburn symptoms, you know that your stomach is producing sufficient amounts.

Unfortunately, this is usually not the case. For many people their HcL is too low and they can supplement up to 5,000mg with a meal. This will provide the digestive support they need to properly break down food without causing post meal discomfort. Supplementing with HcL should be short term, as your stomach gets stronger, you will likely need less dosage as your stomach repairs. Approximately one tablespoon of organic apple cider vinegar (with water) with each meal will also encourage your own stomach acid to be produced and act as a wonderful digestive aid.

NERVES AND DIGESTIVE HEALTH

Our nervous system is made up of more than a billion nerve cells called neurons. They run throughout the body and make connections between our brain and other parts of the body. Having optimal flow of neurons within our nervous system plays a critical role in how our digestive system functions. This is the only fight my chiropractor husband and I continue to battle – What controls our body? Is it our nervous system? or is it our gut? Our gut controls how our nervous system works, and therefore our gut controls our body. He would be delighted that I am backing up his argument in a sense, that if the nerve that controls digestion (our vagus nerve) is cut off, there would be absolutely no movement to this area, causing a condition called gastroparesis. Symptoms of halted digestive activity or gastroparesis include nausea, and vomiting undigested foods hours after eating. Anyone experiencing any communication issue within their body must be properly checked by a licensed Chiropractor. I remember one patient who I was supporting by eliminating food intolerances and through colon hydrotherapy care and who was still suffering from extreme constipation. As a last trial effort I suggested having her spine assessed, wondering if there was something affecting the nerve flow to her bowels. Literally after one adjustment her bowels were now moving daily, and she no longer had issues with constipation. There is no argument here, we need healthy nerve flow, and healthy function of all organs in order for them to create strong immune responses, optimal digestion, and nutrient absorption.

THE GUT OF THE MATTER

Our colon is by far the most important eliminative channel, consisting of approximately 20 feet of small intestine and 6 feet of large intestine.

Within the majority of people, I have found that the bowel is the most underactive organ in the body. The purpose of the small intestine, with its finger-like villi is where the digestion, absorption, and assimilation of foods takes place. The large intestine is divided into four sections; the ascending, transverse, descending, and sigmoid colon. It removes excess water and eliminates your waste from your body. If your bowel is sluggish and underactive, it increases the burden of toxicity within the body causing stress and most likely bowel issues. This stress creates more toxic material that goes into the bloodstream and lymphatic system and then settles in the inherently weak organs and tissues of the body. Organs most affected by bowel underactivity are the lungs and bronchioles, kidneys, skin, liver and lymphatic system. A whole cascade of symptoms occur when these organs are not clean, such as skin issues, more anxiety, and less energy. Toxicity and an overburdened blood stream due to an underactive bowel affects every tissue in the body, and our genetically weak tissues first. For example; ever notice when you get sick all infections seem to go to the lungs? Or chronic kidney infections?

Whether it's an infection in the lungs or kidneys, our whole body will function more effectively once we take care of our gut.

It is critical that we pay attention to when the bowel needs to move, and do not wait. Let the bowel empty entirely. When you ignore the needs of the bowel, interference with other bodily functions eventually will develop. Ignoring the call of nature too often can cause a loss of sensitivity of nerve endings in the bowel, making you unaware of the time for elimination and ultimately leading to frequent constipation. On the other hand, never force or strain a movement. This could cause a rupture, hemorrhoids, or other rectal problems. Hemorrhoids are varicose veins that are caused by too much force and strain placed upon your rectum by stool. Appendicitis can be another result of chronic constipation.

The appendix is a small fingerlike projection that branches off the large intestine at the lower right-hand side of the abdomen. It is primarily lymphoid tissue, which provides a defense against local infection. People who become afflicted with appendicitis have often been constipated for years.

When the colon becomes blocked and clogged in the area of the appendix with old waste material that has not been eliminated, the appendix can easily become infected.

Keeping your colon happy

The colon is the most important elimination channel for us to take care of. Here are some insights to how you can keep your colon clean. High fiber diets can help a great deal. Raw or lightly steamed vegetables and fresh fruits provide good fiber. All foods that are yellow in color are natural laxatives, particularly good for the colon. These foods are high in magnesium, which directly benefits the peristaltic action of the bowel. Yellow squash, peaches, pears, are also great for keeping the colon well. Whole grains also contain a large amount of fiber which absorbs water, and swells up, which again, helps keep the colon clean.

Another way you can cleanse your colon is with alfalfa tablets. They are high in chlorophyll and fiber and acidophilus which puts good bacteria in the intestinal tract. Chlorella powder or tablets are excellent foods for nourishing the good bacteria and cleansing the colon. Omega 3's are important for relieving inflammation. Fish of many kinds are rich sources of omega 3 fatty acids. Prunes and prune juice can also be helpful in maintaining regularity or relieving constipation. Cascara is a gentle, natural laxative, however, when used frequently and often can weaken the bowel musculature and create dependency.

Try to avoid coffee as much as possible and teas that contain caffeine. A good substitute in the morning is a cup of warm water or herbal tea. That NEED for caffeine in the morning is a sign other organ systems are off, and needing to be looked in to. Constipation can have many causes and can lead to many other ailments. Its most frequent cause is dehydration – failure to drink enough water will most certainly turn up as constipation. We all need to drink eight to twelve 8 ounce glasses of water each day. It takes time and determination to develop new eating, drinking, and living habits, but for the sake of colon health, it is well worthwhile.

Our gut and microbiome

Another big part of our gut is our microbiome,

a system that has become increasingly more researched regarding its utmost importance in our immune system. It is responsible for absorbing nutrients, and producing vitamin K, and folate. Short chain fatty acids are also produced here, they are the main nutrient source for our colon and reduce overall inflammation in our body. Another main function is producing serotonin, also known as our "happy hormone". We have trillions of good bacteria that help fight off the bad bacteria. A famous doctor named Bernard Jenson stated, "All diseases start in the gut." In other words, without a healthy gut, there is no way our body can fight any disease effectively.

There are many things that damage our bodies microbiome, such as taking pharmaceutical drugs or antibiotics, and high cortisol (stress), processed foods, preservatives, herbicides/pesticides, and environmental toxicity. When the gut flora contains an imbalance, not enough good vs bad, we call this dysbiosis. This dysbiosis has been linked to a whole host of metabolic issues including insulin resistance, obesity, inflammatory bowel disease and cancer. Below is a list of changes you can implement right away to directly impact your gut fighting power and longevity.

1. Try natural alternatives prior to using a medication. For example, if you have a headache, maybe you are dehydrated? More water could help, or maybe you have magnesium glycinate and vitamin B deficiency. Before grabbing a pain killer (tylenol, advil etc.), look into possible nutritional deficiencies that may be causing this headache.

2. It is a fact that antibiotics kill off our healthy gut bacteria, but so do natural agents like colloidal silver, and oil of oregano. If you have ever taken conventional or natural antibiotics, be sure to supplement with high dosage multi-strain **probiotics** for at least 3 months post use to help rebuild balance.

3. Boost prebiotic levels. They are a type of fiber that promotes the growth of friendly gut bacteria. For example lentils, chickpeas, beans, artichokes, leeks and onions are high in prebiotic fiber and happen to be delicious.

4. Go organic. Each year there are revised versions

of the "clean 15" foods that are least saturated with herbicide and pesticide use. Look into the foods that must be eaten organic, in general, they will be the foods with thin skins that easily absorb these chemicals like berries and celery and unlike fruits and vegetables with harder and denser skins like avocado and bananas.

5. Ditch the fast food. We know you are what you eat, so don't be cheap, fast, and of poor quality. Think of all quick (pre-made) foods as nutrient-less, and full of preservatives which further the abnormal flora in our guts.

6. Avoid environmental toxicities by wearing a mask outside and live in a bubble. (Just kidding!) Avoid the things in our control, for example start in your home. Furniture, clothing, and other household products are highly laden with chemicals. When purchasing anything for your home, including paints, check for low VOC content (Volatile Organic Compounds), and let them air out prior to bringing them into your home. Also cleaning supplies, ditch the chemicals and use lemon, vinegar and

your favourite essential oils instead. All these toxicities not only wreak havoc on your gut, but will present as irritations, and potential future allergic reactions.

Taking these initiates will do wonders to your gut microbiome. If you want to have an exact measure of what the good versus bad bacteria load ratio is in your gut, a comprehensive stool analysis is recommended. This is discussed further in the testing section of this guide.

INSULIN RESISTANCE

When we talk about ultimate digestion, it's important to know how we absorb food nutrients into the body. After sugars are ingested in the form of carbohydrates or sugar; the pancreas (more specifically, cells called beta cells within the pancreas) release a hormone called insulin. Insulin acts as a transporter which carries the sugar to the body's cells and allows the sugar to be absorbed by the cells. If insulin is constantly being spiked in the body, the cells become tired and therefore they move slower and can become exhausted. Imagine a garage door opener – if you constantly push the button to open the door every few minutes, eventually, the battery will stop working, and the garage door will not open. This term is called "insulin resistance." With insulin resistance, sugar can no longer be absorbed by the cells effectively and instead of being absorbed and used as energy, sugar starts to be stored in other areas of the body like your blood, muscles, liver, and fat cells.

If we have insulin resistance, we feel thirsty and hungry, even after a meal. Our cells are essentially starving because the insulin is not allowing our cells to absorb the sugar that is in our systems and unbeknownst, our brain tells our body that we need more sugar, even though this is the last thing our body actually needs.

Sugar is also transported to the liver and muscles in the form of glycogen. When the glycogen stores are full, insulin will also take sugar out of the bloodstream, and the body will convert it and store it as excess fat.

The main purpose of insulin is to keep the blood sugar level from getting too high and moving excess carbohydrates or sugars out of the bloodstream where they can be stored into the tissues for later use. In our society we eat a lot of white flour, refined sugars, white rice, and other starchy foods. These foods are triggering this excess insulin production which causes us to gain weight because it is being stored as fat. When we have a diet that is full of processed sugar and carbohydrates, our body will constantly have to produce insulin to keep up. We can measure the sugar content by understanding the glycemic index (GI) of certain foods. The higher the sugar or glycemic index, the more insulin our body will produce and release. Foods with a low GI trigger less insulin production.

When our body encounters constant spikes of insulin, our cells start the process of becoming insulin resistant. When there is more inflammation going on in the tissues, we cannot absorb critical nutrients, which leads down the path of further resistance to insulin. When the cells stop absorbing insulin they cannot absorb sugar. This causes a large amount of sugar to float aimlessly within your bloodstream and your blood sugar level can become too high. As a result, high blood sugar levels affect brain function, as well as the functionality of all other organs in the body.

The high insulin levels also contribute to chronic disease processes like cancer because high insulin levels interfere with production of prostaglandins (an anti-inflammatory response). High insulin is also a growth stimulator which is found to be high in most cancers.

Our body is made up of trillions of cells that contain all the material necessary for life. Cells manage a wide range of functions: growing, moving, and detoxing. We have over 70 trillion cells that make up tissues, and these tissues make up our organs. Each cell has a lifespan of 1-2 months. Every 24 hours our body replaces an entire layer of tissue, getting rid of the old cells, and replacing them with new cells. That means that our bodies are producing billions of cells daily. Cellular nutrients come in different forms including sugars, proteins, and fats. In order to provide a cell with energy, these digested food molecules have to pass through the cell membrane where over a thousand chemical reactions occur.

Each cell membrane has a gate on its receptor where messages attach themselves and these gates have to be opened for these messages to get in. Who knew insulin was such an essential part of our livelihood and would be the key to opening and allowing nutrient absorption to our cells. But the important lesson here is even insulin needs to be balanced in order to help your body function properly.

THE IMMUNE SYSTEM

When it comes to how our body fights microbes, and abnormal cells, it's important to know what makes up the immune system. This system consists mainly of white blood cells. They are classified into groups: neutrophils, lymphocytes, eosinophils, monocytes, and basophils, and this is based on their function and how they come together to fight infections and disease. We want to do everything in our power to keep this system strong and healthy, from fighting off the common cold, improving healing time, preventing infection, and the most important battle- fighting cancer.

These white blood cells are constantly

circulating around our lymphatic system, scavenging for bacteria, viruses, and anything foreign in the body. We are more likely to get sick when these immune cells are low. Some other cells in the immune system are macrophages, or white blood cells that eat large foreign particles. These cells are called "natural killer cells" (NK) and they are your immune system's first responders and they will quickly destroy harmful cells. B cells produce antibodies that fight infection, and dendritic cells and also activate T cells. So, what would cause these cells to weaken and not work at their best? The answer is simple: chronic stress, poor diet, lack of sleep, smoking, and nutritional deficiencies. I know that after reading this book you will feel encouraged to do everything you can to eliminate these immune suppressors, and give your body the relief and strength it needs to fight the battle of a lifetime.

THE LYMPHATIC SYSTEM

We all have an amazing network of lymphatic vessels and organs that carry fluid called lymph throughout our body. Our spleen is our main lymphatic organ, that stores white blood cells, and filters out toxicity within blood. Lymphatic glands and nodes are found along the neck, spine, lungs, the under arm, groin, abdomen, and legs. Lymph glands make up a system that is like a garbage and debris collection service that works all around the body, and its main function is to move and transfer fluid, and this makes up our immune system.

When you are sick, and feel the nodes in your neck, you are feeling immune cells called lymphocytes concentrated in the lymph nodes. So the next time you have an inflamed area, trust your body is doing its work, and that it is actively trying to fight any infection that should not be there. When we have chronic infections, it is common mainstream practice for these lymphatic tissues like our tonsils and appendix to be removed. These pockets of garbage collectors serve a purpose, so removing them eliminates our "warning sign" that something is off in the body. Just like if you had burglars constantly breaking into your car, and decided that taking that annoying loud alarm system away would solve the problem, we all know it wouldn't. It's ignoring the real problem.

You need a stronger army to fight those burglars away so they don't stand a chance. By boosting your immune system that is the exact approach you would be taking; you would be encouraging immune cells to fight stronger. Seventy percent of our immune cells are located in your gut, which is why so much attention is directed towards gut health. When your goal is to fight cancer effectively, focusing on gut health will only strengthen your immune health, creating a systemic effect to make you stronger overall and providing your body the ability to fight anything else that tries to bring your system down.

Homework for ultimate immune and gut health[2]

1. **Make a conscious effort to relax when you eat.**

   Turn off your phone, turn off the TV. Sit down and spend some quality time focusing on your breath, slowing your chew and giving your body time to properly digest.

2. **Increase foods and drinks that feed your colonocytes (cells of the colon)**

   Food examples: Papaya, liquid chlorophyll, chlorella, prunes, figs, spinach, sun-dried olives, chard, celery, kale, beet greens, whey, shredded beet, watercress, yogurt, rice bran, kefir, psyllium husks, sauerkraut, and kimchi

   Drink examples: parsley juice, papaya juice, chlorophyll, carrot juice, potato peeling broth, whey, prune juice, water with bentonite clay, 2-3 liters of plain water daily (juices and teas don't count), kombucha

3. **Dump all the processed sugar in your house.**
   Look at it like a drug. If it's around you, you will likely eat it. So get rid of those temptations that only bring you down!

4. **See your Naturopathic Doctor to check for mineral deficiencies, and supplement if not getting adequate amounts into your diet.**
   Common mineral deficiencies are: magnesium,

sodium, chlorine, potassium, iron, sulfur, copper, silicon, zinc, and iodine

5. **Incorporate colon enhancing herbs into each day.**

   Examples: alfalfa, aloe vera, peppermint, slippery elm, cayenne, burdock, comfrey, ginger, fennel, anise. As a last resort, add cascara sagrada as needed to encourage daily bowel movements.

Step 3: Understanding Why Cancer Grows

Once you understand the biology (the study of living organisms) and physiology (the study of how these living organisms function within your body) of your disease, you can begin to work on your system metabolically (the study of living organisms and their metabolism).

The truth is, all diseases kick start a process that your body reacts to in order to maintain balance. For example: high blood pressure. We label "hypertension" as a disease. We need to realize that the body, and in all its intelligence, knows that the arteries are clogged and inflamed and in order to get the right amount of blood to flow through every organ, the body has to increase the pressure. Instead of looking at that process as a disease, it is actually working as a cure to the problem. Therefore, taking medication to "lower blood pressure" does not fix the underlying issue that there are clogged arteries and the sole reason as to why the heart is needing to work harder in the first place. Cutting out a cancerous tumor does provide immediate care, but does not give a long term solution. We need to understand what caused it to grow in the first place.

CANCER AS A SYSTEMIC DISEASE

Cancer is never localized to one area of the body. Yes, it may appear in only one place, but your mind, gut, nervous system, and immune system – the whole body – affects its growth. Taking a deeper look at any imbalance and a deeper look into your body's biochemistry will help you understand why cancer grew in the first place, and what you can do to prevent and limit its growth.

There are many theories as to why cancer is initiated in the body. For many years, research has been done to find "the cure for cancer." Instead of finding a single drug or "cure" it's time we look at the body as a whole, and take a metabolic approach.

Metabolic Approach

I want to focus on the things that are in our control to change. Explained using the metabolic approach, we can begin to understand why abnormal cells grow in the body. In 1931, Dr. Otto Warburg won a Nobel prize for the theory that cancer was essentially abnormal cell metabolism, specifically in the mitochondria within the cells.[1] The mitochondria can be summarized as the main energy-producing part of the cell and they are all damaged within cancerous cells.[2]

Dr. Warburg also found that cancer occurs when any cell is denied sixty percent of its oxygen, and the main function in the mitochondria is to produce oxygen. Cancer is the final event in the body's cell cycle. When those cells lose the ability to use oxygen they go into a default mode of energy production, called "fermentation", as a result of down-regulating all their antioxidant enzymes. There are several things that are actually proven to damage our cells' mitochondria and their oxygen-producing abilities, including toxicity and stress on the body. Some examples of toxicity are tobacco smoke, alcohol, radiation, obesity, and other inflammatory triggers, such as mold, bacteria, and viruses.[3] Over exposure to sunlight, along with age, have also been shown to decrease the health of our mitochondria. Eliminating these toxic habits is a critical step to ultimate wellness. It is also exciting that many of the things mentioned for healthy digestive and immune function are the exact practices that support health mitochondrial function – such as meditation, proper sleep, fasting, low sugar foods, and eliminating inflammatory triggers. As well, additional testing will provide you a deeper understanding of what may be damaging your mitochondria on a cellular level, and as you keep reading you will likely come upon mention of advanced treatments that will help resolve this damage.

Genetics?

Research has found that up to 90% of cancers can be attributed to environmental factors.[4] This also means, up to 90% of cancers can **actually be prevented** by understanding how to implement strategies to diminish these environmental triggers.

During initial assessments with patients, I do like to understand family history, because genetics needs to be considered when looking at cancer growth. However, I put emphasis on the fact that we have so much power to change the outcome, since inherited genetic mutations are only 5-10% of all cancers.[5]

Epigenetics

Even if we were born with a genetic imprint

predisposing us to cancer, it is exciting to know that several lifestyle factors can modify whether these genes turn on or not! The study of epigenetics helps us understand how DNA is regulated, and what in our power can control these on/off switches. The most known factors that modify epigenetic patterns include tobacco, alcohol, pollutants, stress, poor diet, obesity, night shifts, and physical activity.[6] With this being said, you are five times more likely to have cancer if you have a genetic predisposition to it.[7] Which is why studying genes in relation to cancer growth is so important.

The two main genes responsible for controlling our cells growth and division are called oncogenes and "tumor suppressor" genes. Oncogenes are like pressing the gas accelerator in your car, when they're turned on, these genes are activated. Tumor suppressor genes (TSG) are the opposite. Abnormal cell growth happens when these genes are inactivated and turned off. TSG genes slow down how the cells divide, repair our DNA, and tell cells when to die (a process called apoptosis, or programmed cell death).[8]

This is the exact problem with cancer cells.

When there is a mutation or damage in a TSG, typically acquired from ultraviolet (UV) radiation, tobacco, viruses, and/or age, the onset of abnormal cells continue to divide and lose the signal for programmed death. The most common TSG known in breast cancer are BRCA1 and BRCA2 genes.[9] You have likely heard of them as *breast cancer genes*. If you have a mutation in one of these genes, you have an increased risk of developing breast cancer, but not everyone with this gene will actually develop it. This is the target of many conventional treatment protocols being the focus on the abnormal genes that are being expressed. A very powerful realization is that we have so much control in how these genes are being expressed. Understanding carcinogens, aka the agents that have been scientifically proven to cause cancer in these cells is critical information and knowledge that you need to understand so you are able to make environmental changes to prevent these abnormal cells from growing in the body.

Our exposure to toxicity and various stressors on the body which cause inflammation are the main reason these genes become mutated and get turned on. Understanding our defense mechanisms will help us understand why these stressors affect some of us and not others.

Have you ever wondered why some people can smoke their entire life, eat like crap, and never develop cancer, whereas someone else could be doing *everything right*, and they get a cancer diagnosis? It just doesn't seem fair! How your body deals with stress and eliminates waste, both physically and mentally, is a critical part of it.

We must always look at the entire body and how it functions, including digestive, spiritual, and psychological stress, immunity, bodily alignment, muscle tone, and posture, which also play a big role in our nervous system, circulation and lymphatic function. All our organ systems, including the immune system, speak to one another. If there are any misalignments, it will absolutely affect how our body is able to fight any disease, especially breast cancer.

It is exciting to understand that in the following chapters you will learn all the ways you can enhance your body's ability to dissolve this free radical damage and dispose of toxicity more effectively so these genes don't continue to wreak havoc on your system. Also in Chapter 4, "Additional Testing", you will understand why thorough testing is needed to look beyond the genes you were born with, and putting that knowledge into an action plan to fight cancer effectively.

Hormonal Triggers

Breast cancer can be divided into a few categories based on what feeds its growth. Estrogen and progesterone are the most common. When someone is estrogen-positive, it's important to understand that there are a few versions of estrogen and not all are bad. If you have estrogen-positive cancer, you shouldn't fear this hormone. Consider its role in your body. Estrogen supports bone formation and growth, it increases in vaginal lubrication, it supports metabolism, your protein formation, and your organ systems.

If you have estrogen dominant breast cancer, the very thought of estrogen may create fear and anxiety, and these emotions have the potential ability to stimulate your cancer growth. Understanding estrogen in all forms will help put your mind at ease.

You need to know that there are three different types of estrogens as a result of estrone being metabolized in the liver. 2-OH-estrone metabolite is the most protective against breast cancer.[10] The higher the level in your body, the lesser the risk of breast cancer. 4-OH-estrone, and 16-OH estrone both have DNA mutating effects that can lead to abnormal and uncontrolled cell growth, which is a precursor to cancer.[11]

After testing, which is further explained in the "Advanced Testing" chapter, you can take proactive measures to balance hormones. This means supporting your body in eliminating the harmful estrogen metabolites, and enhancing the protective ones. When working in the clinic, I hear that there is an issue with how you metabolize estrogens or when I hear you say you've been diagnosed with fibroids and have raging premenstrual syndrome and have intense irritability throughout the month, I know instinctively that there is a problem! Women are predisposed to think it's a normal condition of being born a female to have raging hormones! Let me tell you, it's not! Our liver plays a huge role in this process of estrogen balancing, it inactivates and excretes these bad estrogens in a process called phase 1 and phase 2 detoxification. If the liver is overwhelmed and not fed the correct nutrients, it will not be able to break down these estrogens effectively. My favourite supplements used to support excess estrogens in the body are milk thistle, indole-3-carbinol, calcium-d-glucarate, dandelion, turmeric and DIM. Supporting estrogen metabolism is fantastic, however we also want to be aware of the various sources that we may be exposing ourselves to that exacerbate the issue.

Dirty Estrogens

When it comes to any estrogen based condition, whether its breast cancer, fibroids, premenstrual syndrome, the term xenoestrogen is also important to understand. These types of estrogens are chemicals that mimic natural estrogen in your body, but come from a foreign source. These fake estrogens are able to throw hormone balance off, giving them the term endocrine disruptors. They have the ability to stimulate how cancer grows in the body.

This is a list of all the estrogenic chemicals that you need to be aware of so you can eliminate them from your life.

List of Estrogenic Chemicals to be **ELIMINATED** from your life:[12]

- Alkylphenol
- Atrazine (weedkiller)
- Butylated hydroxyanisole / BHA (food preservative)
- Chlorine and chlorine by-products
- Bisphenol A (monomer for polycarbonate plastic and epoxy resin; antioxidant in plasticizers)
- Dichlorodiphenyldichloroethylene (one of the breakdown products of DDT)
- DEHP (plasticizer for PVC)
- Methoxychlor (insecticide)
- 4-Methylbenzylidene camphor (4-MBC) (sunscreen lotions)
- Metalloestrogens (a class of inorganic xenoestrogens)
- Polychlorinated biphenyls / PCBs (in electrical oils, lubricants, adhesives, paints)
- Pentachlorophenol (general biocide and wood preservative)

- Polychlorinated biphenyls / PCBs (in electrical oils, lubricants, adhesives, paints)
- Dieldrin (insecticide)
- DDT (insecticide)
- Nonylphenol and derivatives (industrial surfactants; emulsifiers for emulsion polymerization; laboratory detergents; pesticides)
- Parabens (methylparaben, ethylparaben, propylparaben and butylparaben commonly used as preservatives in personal care products)
- Endosulfan (insecticide)
- Phenosulfothiazine (a red dye)
- Erythrosine / FD&C Red No. 3
- Phthalates (plasticizers)
- Ethinylestradiol (combined oral contraceptive pill)
- Lindane / hexachlorocyclohexane (insecticide)
- Propyl gallate
- Heptachlor (insecticide)

Guidelines To Minimize Your Exposure To Xenoestrogens:[13]

- Choose chlorine-free products and unbleached paper products.
- Use glass or ceramics whenever possible to store food.
- Don't refill plastic water bottles.
- Avoid creams and cosmetics that have toxic chemicals and estrogenic ingredients such as parabens and stearal konium chloride.
- Do not leave plastic containers, especially your drinking water, in the sun. *If a plastic water container has heated up significantly, throw it away - do not drink the water.
- Whenever possible, choose organic foods.
- Avoid freezing water in plastic bottles to drink later.
- Buy hormone free meats and dairy products to avoid hormones and pesticides.
- Buy food grown locally and in season, organic if possible.
- Use chlorine free tampons, menstrual pads, toilet paper, paper towel, coffee filters, etc.
- Peel non-organic fruits and vegetables.
- Reduce the use of plastics whenever possible.

- Use chemical free, biodegradable laundry and household cleaning products whenever possible.
- Do not microwave food in plastic containers.
- Use chemical free soaps and toothpastes.
- Avoid the use of plastic wrap to cover food for storing or microwaving.
- Avoid all pesticides, herbicides, and fungicides.
- Minimize your exposure to nail polish and nail polish removers.
- Use naturally based fragrances, such as essential oils.
- Be aware of noxious gas such as from copiers and printers, carpets, fiberboards, and at the gas pump.
- Minimize X-rays whenever possible.
- Read the labels on condoms and diaphragm gels.
- Use filtered water to drink and bathe in to avoid chlorine.

Even if you do not have estrogen positive cancer, you still want to avoid these sources and balance estrogen since in general, estrogen stimulates proliferation in the body. On a cellular level any excess or inflammatory process will further imbalance and negatively affect cancer growth.

HOW DOES SUGAR IMPACT CANCER?

There is a common misunderstanding regarding how sugar affects cancerous growth and many oncologists say there is no issue at all to keeping your regular sugar habits in your diet. On the contrary; I want to explain why keeping sugar in your diet is a horrible idea.

The issue with sugar comes down to insulin resistance. As previously mentioned, cells in our muscles, fat, and liver do not respond to the insulin that carries in the sugar to be transferred into energy. This is also the reason why hundreds of thousands of people in North America are diagnosed with type-II diabetes. If sugar cannot be absorbed by your cells, then the sugar accumulates into the blood (causing high blood sugar), and your pancreas will produce more and more insulin to respond to the higher sugar levels in the blood. Insulin is a growth hormone, which means: the more insulin you produce because of your insulin resistance, the more your cells will grow and replicate. This is the exact process that stimulates cancer growth.[14] There is a specific test available that can tell if your cancer is growing because of insulin (detailed in the testing section).

THE WARBURG EFFECT

The Warburg effect is a phenomenon which further explains how mitochondria, the energy center of our cells, is involved with cancer. As discussed earlier, our bodies heavily rely on oxygen to create energy. We call this process "aerobic respiration," during which our mitochondria uses oxygen to make energy. This is the most healthy and efficient way for our bodies to create energy.

If these mitochondria are damaged in any way, our cells are so intelligent that they will start making energy (ATP) from another (much less) efficient process, called "fermentation" or *glycolysis*. Our body creates eighteen times more healthy energy (ATP) from aerobic respiration compared to glycolysis. Otto Warburg's studies found that cancer cells heavily rely on glycolysis, and through this process cancer cells fuel themselves with large amounts of sugar compared to normal healthy cells.[15]

Sugar, Insulin, and Growth Hormone

To further understand how sugar affects cell growth and its relationship to cancer, I want to explain a type of dwarfism called Laron Syndrome. Within the Laron Syndrome population there is a high sensitivity to insulin, and a low level of growth hormone, and to further support the above point about sugar and cell growth, the fascinating thing about individuals who have Laron Syndrome is that they have virtually no diabetes and no cancer present.[16] How interesting, right!

Another fact we know about sugar and cancer is the ingestion of a sugar derivative during a PET scan. This sugar is used to locate and light up any cancer cell activity in the body. We cannot deny the fact that cancer cells have a very different reaction to sugar than normal healthy cells do. You controlling sugar intake and reversing insulin resistance will make a drastic difference on cancer initiation and growth that can be controlled on a cellular level.

One of the best ways to reverse insulin resistance is through intermittent fasting and ketogenic diets – both discussed in the fasting chapter.

On a clinical note, I find it interesting how almost every person/ patient I see with cancer undoubtedly all experience sugar cravings. Sugar is like a drug to them and they feel they need it in their life in order to suppress 'the need' which is very similar to addictions. The need for sugar is not always through the eating of processed desserts and candy, but also in the form of fruits, wine, and other carbohydrates. This is a huge red flag to me that insulin resistance is present. Increasing how much fats and proteins you have in your diet will help prevent sugar cravings, but really the most effective thing to do is get all of those sugary sweet temptations out of sight. Literally think of it like an addiction to crack and hopefully this connection will help you rid your home of it. The best way to start reversing insulin resistance and balance how your body uses sugar is to drastically minimize its intake.

Now that you are likely feeling down and feeling like you can't eat anything that sits presently in your kitchen cupboards in order to starve cancer out of your system, in the next chapter, I want to emphasize the foods that you can and should eat to help fight cancer more effectively.

Step 4: Foods That Fight Cancer

"Illnesses do not come out of the blue. They are developed from small daily sins against nature. When enough sins have accumulated, illnesses will suddenly appear." – Hippocrates

THE POWER OF FOOD

Now that you know about cancer's growth and know what not to eat and what toxins and chemicals that you should eliminate from your daily life, you might be wondering, *"What should I eat in order to help my health while diminishing my cancer cells?"* Everything that you ingest should be viewed as *feeding cancer cells or fighting cancer cells*.

When it comes to food we have so much power to redirect these cells and start a chain reaction to create strength within our body. With all the fad diets out there, how do we know which one is the right one? More importantly, how do we know which diet is the right one for someone with breast cancer? Our bodies need the right balance of vitamins and minerals, carbohydrates, proteins, and fats in order to function and stay alive. If any of these components are missing over a long period of time, our body will take a hit, and will become tired and lack immune function. Let's dive into nutrition starting with the basic understanding of what your foods are.

Carbs, Proteins, Fat

Carbohydrates, proteins, and fats are all types of macronutrients, and each is critical to have in your diet for strength and survival. When you ingest protein, your body breaks it down into amino acids. Amino acids are the building blocks of your immune system. They build and repair the tissue and muscles in your body, and they can also be used for producing energy. Animal sources will provide the highest amount of protein per serving; however this may not be the healthiest way for everyone to achieve adequate levels.

For example: Japanese-American females who are raised eating Westernized diets, have a higher rate of breast cancer when compared to Japanese women who are raised eating more traditional Japanese foods. Even within the country of Japan, affluent women who eat meat daily have an 8.5 times higher risk of breast cancer than women who are impoverished and rarely or never eat meat protein.[1] Healthy and alternative to meat proteins recommended for all women with breast cancer include non-GMO soy, nuts, and beans.

You can view carbohydrates as the foods that are quick energy sources. This is why when you're tired or need something to eat quickly, you typically reach for carbs, i.e. crackers, chips or breads. Depending on which carbohydrates you choose, they can have positive effects and be an excellent source of fiber helping you carry waste out of the body and regulating bowel movements. Too many carbohydrates though, will again, spike sugar levels, leading to insulin resistance and hormone imbalances. Healthy and recommended sources of carbohydrates include many types of vegetables (excluding white potatoes), beans, peas, lentils, nuts, and seeds.

For years, many fad diets tried to make people refrain from eating fat, but we quickly learned that low-fat diets result in intake of more sugar and carbohydrates, leading to a whole cascade of health issues, such as obesity and diabetes. Therefore, over the past few years, the ketogenic and paleo diets have thrived. Since all the cells in our body are surrounded by a fat layer, ingesting healthy sources of mono and polyunsaturated fats will boost how our body communicates and functions, including balancing hormones, keeping us feeling full, promoting healthy skin, and improving brain health; just to name a few positive impacts of eating fats. Fats are also critical to help absorb certain vitamins, such as Vitamin A, D, E and K. It's the saturated fat and trans-fat that we need to stay away from and these can be found in deep-fried foods. These types of fat have the opposite effect on our body, which causes plaque buildup in our arteries, making our cells rigid, and preventing nutrients from being absorbed. This is another reason for why animal products that are high in fat should be avoided. Consumption of deep fried foods, and fatty animal meats will drive production of hormones, which in turn, promotes growth of cancer cells in hormone-sensitive organs such as the breasts.[2]

Meat is devoid of the protective effects of fiber, antioxidants, phytochemicals, and other helpful nutrients, and it contains high concentrations of saturated fat and potentially carcinogenic compounds, which may increase one's risk of developing breast cancer. Examples of healthy fats that regulate hormones and strengthen your body include nuts, hemp seeds, and chia seeds, avocado, and olive oil. You can also consume more foods with omega-fatty acids, such as wild salmon, tuna, halibut, mackerel, sardines, and herring, and again, more nuts and seeds.

VEGETARIANISM

A twenty year long study completed in China describes how choosing low fat proteins, and vegetarian eating habits has been scientifically proven as the best diet for fighting breast cancer.[3] This study focussed on nutrition and risk for diseases, including cancer, in one of the longest and most comprehensive studies ever. The study stated that a diet with animal protein and dairy is a risk factor for cancer. Concluding that the whole-food, plant-based diets decrease this risk. Dr. T. Colin Campbell Ph.D says that in multiple, peer-reviewed animal studies, researchers discovered that they could actually turn the growth of cancer cells on and off by raising and lowering doses of casein, the main protein found in cow's milk.[4] Another main reason for this finding is that animal meat is pro-inflammatory. Many animal meats are also full of hormones and drugs which cause unforeseen stress on your body when eaten. Grass fed animals are safer, due to a more favorable omega-3 to omega-6 fat ratio. Omega-3 brings down inflammation in the body and supports health immune function. Omega-3 can be found high in foods like seaweed, algae, chia seeds, hemp, flax seeds, walnuts, edamame, soy and kidney beans. Foods high in omega-6 include corn, safflower and sunflower oil, meat and poultry.

There are also supplementary options like vegetarian oils that provide high omega-3's from algae, to further ensure a balanced ratio of these different types of fats. However, to touch on both sides, on the contrary to all the good and healthy, one of the issues with vegan or vegetarian diets is the tendency to be higher in carbohydrates and sugars, which can drive the inflammatory process and also stimulate cortisol and throw off hormone balance.

Because I place a high level of importance on low inflammatory and plant based diets, I have included meal plans to remove the guessing out of what should be eaten each day. These plans can be strictly followed or generally but will help guide you to eating with the purpose of balancing hormones and fighting cancer cells.

THE GLYCEMIC INDEX (GI)

The glycemic index puts a number to the amount of carbohydrates and sugar found in a source of food and how quickly the sugar is released into your bloodstream (this is the important part). When you have cancer, you want to eat foods that are the **lowest** on the glycemic index, meaning, foods with less of a sugar load and those foods that will limit sugar spikes. The most important thing to understand when it comes to cancer is how sugar can wreak havoc on your body, causing extreme inflammation and throwing hormones off balance. Cancer cells love sugar and sugar proliferates cancerous growth.[5]

However, when thinking about sugary foods we usually jump right to the sweet desserts we eat. What we forget to consider is the carbohydrates we eat that ultimately turn into sugar as soon as they are ingested. A bowl of pasta or a bowl of ice cream...

it turns into the same stuff. All the breads, pastas, and even starchy vegetables we eat, put a high sugar load onto the body. When you eliminate these foods with a low glycemic diet, it reduces your cancerous growth by controlling insulin and insulin-like growth factors. If you find you crave sugar all the time, you should look into the source; knowing whether or not you have blood sugar issues or are insulin resistant is the first step. Following a low glycemic diet will help cure this sugar craving over time. Below is a generalized list of common foods with its associated glycemic index. With cancer you want to choose foods that have a lower glycemic index (GI) rating, which will elicit a lower the blood sugar response. This chart can be deceiving, since next, we must understand the difference between glycemic index of foods, versus its glycemic load (GL).

LOW GLYCEMIC INDEX (55 or less) [6]

Fruits

Apples (120g)	40
Apple juice (250g)	39
Apricots, dried (60g)	32

Bananas (120g)   47

Fruit cocktail (120g)   55

Grapefruit (120g)   25

Grapes (120g)   43

Mangoes (120g)   51

Oranges, raw (120g)   48

Peaches, canned (120g)   52

Pineapple (120g)   51

Plums (120g)   53

Strawberries (120g)   40

Vegetables

Carrot juice (250g)   43

Carrots, raw (80g)   35

Corn, sweet (80g)   55

Lima beans (150g)   32

Parsnips (80g)   52

Potato (150g)   54

Tomato soup (250g)   38

Grains and Breads

Barley (150g)   22

Basmati rice (150g)   52

Bran cereal (30g)	43
Brown rice (50g)	50
Bulgur wheat (150g)	46
Chickpeas (150g)	36
Instant noodles (180g)	52
Instant oatmeal (25g)	50
Mixed grain bread (30g)	52
Oat bran bread (30g)	44
Rye kernel bread (30g)	41
Rye flour bread (30g)	50
Water crackers (25g)	53
White rice, boiled (150g)	47

Nuts and Legumes

Black beans (150g)	30
Butter beans (150g)	36
Cashews (50g)	25
Kidney beans (150g)	29
Kidney beans, canned (150g)	52
Lentils, canned (150g)	42
Split peas, yellow, boiled (150g)	25

Dairy and Alternatives

Skim milk (250g)	32
Soy milk (250g)	43

Snacks and Sweets

Blueberry muffin (60g)	50
Cake, pound (50g)	38
Corn chips (50g)	42
Hummus (30g)	6
Icecream, full-fat, vanilla (50g)	38
Icecream, low-fat, vanilla (50g)	49
Oatmeal cookies (25g)	54
Snickers (60g)	43
Sponge cake (63g)	46
Strawberry jam (30g)	51
Sushi (100g)	55

THE GLYCEMIC LOAD (GL)

The glycemic load (GL) gives a more in depth picture and understanding of how carbohydrates affect our blood sugar level. It is a calculation based on how much carbohydrates are in a specific serving. According to the Harvard School of Public Health, foods rated under 10 for GL are considered low, and these are the foods that are therefore encouraged to eat in order to keep blood sugar levels low.[7]

To understand the difference, let's look at watermelon as an example. It has a GI of 80, being high on the glycemic index, however since it is a very low carbohydrate level, the load is considered to be rated as a 5, making it low on the GL table. Another example is beans. Lentils or pinto beans have a glycemic load that is approximately three times lower than instant mashed potatoes and therefore will not cause large spikes in blood-sugar levels. The ripeness, and preparation method will also affect the GL number. Foods that are high in fiber are also classified to be low on the GL table. These foods include: bran and bran cereals, and legumes such as kidney beans, garbanzo beans (a.k.a. chickpeas), pinto beans, black beans and lentils. Through the foods we choose it is encouraging to know that we can control insulin and insulin like growth factors, reducing our risk of breast cancer by twenty-two percent, just by choosing foods low on the glycemic index as well as having a low glycemic load.[8]

Foods with a low glycemic load of 10 or less:[9]

- Kidney, garbanzo, pinto, soy, and black beans
- Fiber-rich fruits and vegetables, like carrots, green peas, apples, grapefruit, and watermelon
- Cereals made with 100 percent bran
- Lentils
- Cashews and peanuts
- Whole-grain breads like barley, pumpernickel, and whole wheat
- Whole-wheat tortillas
- Tomato juice

Foods with a medium glycemic load of 11 to 19:

- Whole-wheat pasta and some breads
- Oatmeal
- Rice cakes
- Barley and bulgur
- Fruit juices without extra sugar
- Brown rice
- Sweet potato
- Graham crackers

Foods with a high glycemic load of 20 or more:

- High sugar beverages
- Candy
- Sweetened fruit juices
- Couscous
- White rice
- White pasta
- French fries and baked potatoes
- Low-fiber cereals (high in added sugar)
- Macaroni and cheese
- Pizza
- Raisins and dates

CANDIDA AND SUGAR

Having a candida overgrowth will drastically affect how you view sugar. Candida is a yeast that is present in all of us. It makes up our gut microbiome and in small amounts is very healthy and normal. If you have an overgrowth, you also are likely to think about sugar day and night. Not only that, you may feel exhausted, experience brain fog or memory issues, and digestive complaints like gas, bloating and heartburn. In the testing section, you will learn about live blood analysis and the importance of stool testing that can confirm the presence of candida. Candida loves sugar and needs it to replicate, so following a yeast free/anti-candida diet is critical to move forward, and will also help alleviate the other symptoms that go along with it. The cravings for sugar will always be the toughest for the first three to seven days after cutting sugar from your diet; you may even feel withdrawals like headaches, and an exacerbation of low energy, and brain fog, (kind of like you are going through a withdrawal period) but after that, (yes, 'after that'… sorry, I know the common saying is true, "You may feel worse before feeling better!") but trust me, eventually it will be much easier to abstain.[10]

Sugar can literally act as a drug in the body, sending chemicals to your brain that you need more. Like mentioned in the previous chapter, if you keep it out of your sight, it will be much easier to avoid. You can also try agents like caprylic acid, berberine, and oil of oregano to kill off candida overgrowth. If you still crave sugars after following an anti-candida diet, and ingesting anti-candida supplements, you should also look into other sources of why sugar is still on your mind!

ADRENAL (Stress Glands) AND SUGAR

Adrenal health also correlates with sugar cravings, and when your mind and body are exhausted, you will naturally reach for foods higher in sugar and carbs for a quick 'pick me up' and energy boost. These foods break down to sugar quickly in the body, spike cortisol, send glucose to your brain, and give you the short-term fix you were searching for. However, it doesn't end there; when you find yourself reaching for sugar more often, you can assume your body is under more stress than you realize. You are essentially self-medicating to keep yourself going. Still, there is good news – there are much healthier ways to go about this, giving your body the energy you need without creating the inflammatory response time after time. This becomes a vicious cycle that looks like this: stress, high cortisol, low energy, the search for sugary carbohydrates, quick boost of energy, more cortisol, body perceiving more stress, repeat. When you support your adrenal glands properly with the food you eat, you can deal with stress more effectively.

There are specific foods that help rebuild these stress glands, resulting in less cortisol spikes, and therefore less inflammation. Examples of foods that support the adrenal glands (stress glands), are immune-boosting, and also help the body fight cancer are:

- Healthy fats like almonds, walnuts, brazil nuts, all seeds including hemp, chia, sunflower, avocado, and coconut oil.

One of the best ways to regulate sugar, and support adrenal glands are to practice intermittent fasting. This is the practice of only eating foods within a certain time frame of the day to limit excess insulin and cortisol spikes. The instructions of how to do this safely, and its research towards breast cancer remission rates will all be discussed in the "fasting section".

FOODS THAT FIGHT

Foods that fight are foods that strengthen your body, inside and out. Plant foods are high in "phytochemicals," a natural source of chemicals that fight cancer. Lab studies show that they can stimulate immune function, block substances from becoming carcinogenic, reduce inflammation, and slow the growth rate of cancer cells.

Phytochemicals are chemicals found in plants that protect plants against bacteria, viruses, and fungi. Eating large amounts of brightly colored fruits and vegetables (yellow, orange, red, green, white, blue, and purple), whole grains/cereals, and beans containing phytochemicals can decrease the risk of developing certain cancers as well as diabetes, hypertension, and heart disease. The action of phytochemicals varies by color and type of the food. They can act as antioxidants or nutrient protectors, and prevent carcinogens (cancer causing agents) from forming.[11]

Sources of phytochemicals

This is a partial list of phytochemicals that describes which foods you can find and also how they can support your body, beyond cancer.

Allicin is found in onions and garlic. Allicin blocks or eliminates certain toxins from bacteria and viruses. **Anthocyanins** are found in red and blue fruits (such as raspberries and blueberries) and vegetables. They help to slow the aging process, protect against heart disease and tumors, prevent blood clots, and fight inflammation and allergies. **Bioflavonoids** can be found in citrus fruits. These antioxidants quench and destroy free radicals. **Carotenoids** are found in dark yellow, orange, and deep green fruits and vegetables such as tomatoes, parsley, oranges, pink grapefruit, and spinach. They play a therapeutic role in breast cancer. Synthetic beta carotene in a high dose supplement form is not recommended for cancer care. **Flavonoids** are cell regulators and also provide anti-inflammatory, anti-oxidant, and anti-allergy properties. They are found in fruits, vegetables, wine, green tea, onions, apples, kale, and beans. **Indoles** can be found in broccoli, bok choy, cabbage, kale, Brussel sprouts, and turnips (also known as "cruciferous" vegetables). They contain sulfur and activate agents that destroy cancer-causing chemicals. Isoflavones are found in soybeans and soybean products. They decrease risk of recurrent breast cancer, and support healthy bone growth in post menopausal women. **Lignins** are found in flaxseed and whole grain products, reducing cancer risk by supporting healthy estrogen metabolism. **Lutein** are within leafy green vegetables. It may prevent macular degeneration and cataracts as well as reduce the risk of heart disease and breast cancer. **Lycopene** is in tomatoes and tomato products. When cooked, it appears to reduce the risk for cancer and heart attacks, and also reduces IGF-1 stimulation of cancer growth. **Phenolics** are in citrus fruits, fruit juices, cereals, legumes, and oilseeds. They are thought to be extremely powerful, and are studied for a variety of health benefits including slowing the aging process, protecting against heart disease and tumors, and fighting inflammation, allergies, and blood clots. Below is a list of foods high in phytochemicals. Phytochemicals cannot be found in supplements and are only present in food. Foods high in phytochemicals include the following: Broccoli, Berries, Soy nuts, Pears, Turnips, Celery, Carrots, Spinach, Lentils, Cantaloupe, Garlic, Apricots, Onions, Seeds, Soybeans, Green tea, Brussels sprouts, Bok choy, Kale, Red wine, Cabbage, Tomatoes, Apples, Olives [12, 13]

COOKING RULES

To avoid additional burden to your body, it is important to note that it is not always the type of food that you're eating; rather, it is how the food is being prepared. Staying away from foods with pesticides, herbicides, hormones, or animals that were raised on antibiotics and were mainly grain-fed (again, pro-inflammatory) is crucial. Organic foods will also always be a better choice, but how do we know for sure that foods are chemical and pesticide-free? Are the rules and regulations around these foods as strict as we would hope that they would be? The only way to know for sure what your foods are made of is to grow your own garden from organic with non-GMO seeds, but that's a whole different chapter about creating your own whole foods farm.

In general, raw and lightly steamed foods are best for you. Each type of food is affected differently by heat. All *real* (unprocessed) foods contain enzymes to support digestion. They are heat sensitive and can deactivate when exposed to high temperatures. Additionally, many of the vitamins and minerals can become denatured when heated as well.

On the other hand, some foods can benefit from some heat. Tomatoes become more beneficial when heated, because the high heat increases lycopene (which is an antioxidant). In the 2002 issue of the *Journal of Agriculture and Food Chemistry*, Rui Hai Liu, an associate professor of food science at Cornell University, reported that cooking tomatoes increase lycopene within tomatoes by thirty-five percent.

Additionally, carrots, mushrooms, asparagus, cabbage, and peppers contain more antioxidants when boiled or steamed. Carrots and zucchini show increased levels of carotenoid when boiled or steamed.To maximize nutrient levels, it's best to steam vegetables, so they retain their phytochemical compounds that protect against cancer.[14]

Broccoli, however, is best raw; when cooked, broccoli loses its anti-cancer properties. Studies published in the *Journal of Food Chemistry* revealed that after only two minutes, boiled broccoli florets lost at least ninety-five percent of their sulforaphane content, sixty-two percent of their phenolic acid content, twenty-three percent of their glucobrassicin content, and seventeen percent of their glucoraphanin content.[15, 16]

High heat, such as barbequing and deep frying in oil can convert foods to become carcinogenic. This high heat creates free radicals within the food, because this process forms compounds such as heterocyclic amines, polycyclic aromatic hydrocarbons, and acrylamide which are all cancer causing. This can be an issue in vegetarian eating, where vegetables are encouraged. An example of this is with deep fried potatoes which create acrylamide which defeats the purpose of trying to eat more vegetables with the purpose of positive and healthy results. Baking these vegetables would be much healthier and would be a non cancer forming option.

KETOGENIC DIETS

A ketogenic diet follows the same guidelines of low sugar and low carbohydrates. However, the main differentiating factor is that it is rich in fats and includes moderate levels of protein. When following a diet like this, the goal is to get your body into a process called "ketosis". When your body starts producing ketones from fat breakdown it is called "ketosis". The liver's role is to produce these ketones from fat when glucose and insulin levels are low. Ketones are a much cleaner way for our body to create energy. Unlike healthy cells, research has shown that most cancer cells cannot use ketones for energy, so this results in an anti-cancer effect. Also, ketones can be toxic to your cancer cells.

So why are these ketones so powerful against cancer cells? Ketones increase the amount of oxidative stress put onto cancer cells, causing them to go into apoptosis (causing cell death), and they also reduce insulin levels. The keto diet also indirectly fights cancer by reducing one of the main breast cancer stimulating growth hormones called IGF-1. When IGF-1 levels are low, there is less stimulation to promote abnormal cell growth. This type of diet limits these foods which have been shown to increase the hormones that can stimulate cancer growth, which is why it is a diet that has been promoted for cancer patients.

Removing sugars, all grain products, and starchy vegetables, like corn, white potatoes, and most legumes, is important when trying to reach the process of ketosis. Even sugary fruits should be avoided on the keto diet, leaving you to enjoy avocado, lemons, limes, and small amounts or berries to choose from. Supplementing minerals during this diet is necessary since it does leave the body with several deficiencies, such as selenium, copper, and zinc.[17] In general, most people need to have less than fifty grams of net carbohydrates a day (minus how much fiber is in their foods) in order to reach a ketosis state, although some people need as low as twenty to thirty grams to make ketosis possible. This number to reach ketosis will be different for everyone, and the only way of knowing is to measure it.

Measuring Sugar And Ketone Bodies

Just as you would measure blood sugar with glucometers, you can also measure your ketone levels with a hand held device. There is a company called ketomojo.com where you can purchase this device. Another useful way to use this tool is to see what specifically spikes your blood sugar levels, so you are able to stay in ketosis longer. For example, test your first morning blood sugar level and mark down that number. Then drink a cup of black coffee and half an hour later measure blood sugar levels again. If the number stays within a .02 difference then you know you can have coffee within your fasting time without spiking your sugar levels. If there is a larger increase in your sugar levels you will know that black coffee needs to be eliminated in order to get into ketosis effectively. It is a great tool to learn more about your eating habits and which foods you should eliminate from your keto diet while allowing you to know which will be safe for you to eat.

Caution for Ketogenic Diets

Because this diet focuses on high fat consumption, make sure to speak with a knowledgeable health professional prior to starting it. If you have any issues with breaking down fat, there will need to be modifications to this diet. A history of any of the following should lead to modifications within this diet: pancreatitis, active gallbladder disease, high liver enzymes levels, impaired liver function, poor nutritional status, gastric bypass surgery, abdominal tumors causing decreased gastrointestinal motility, history of kidney failure, pregnancy and lactation.

There are also some medications that may be dangerous when starting a ketogenic diet that should be monitored, including anti-seizure medications. They can cause your body to become too acidic, also known as acidosis, and this effect can be even stronger when used in combination with a ketogenic diet. Diuretic medication will also need to be monitored by a medical professional. Ketogenic diets have a natural diuretic effect on the body. Most importantly, if you are undergoing chemotherapy and radiation you should definitely speak to a specialist about how to properly administer a ketogenic diet. Since these types of cancer treatments are extremely toxic to cancer and your body, they can negatively affect your digestive system, and rob the body of critical vitamins and minerals from being absorbed. Going on any extreme change in diet program during this time may also impact your immune system, and liver and kidney function, therefore speaking to an experienced healthcare professional prior to getting started is most definitely necessary.[18]

ESTROGEN FROM FOODS

What's the difference between foods that stimulate estrogen (phyto-estrogen) and those that don't (xeno-estrogen)? When it comes to hormone balance and cancer, the difference is huge and as a cancer patient we want to make sure you understand this difference completely so you can make the right choices for your health in the near future. Phytoestrogens are actually protective against estrogen-fed cancers. Soy, miso, tofu, soy milk and flax seeds actually modulate estrogen receptors. Soy has been given a bad reputation because most people are unaware of what the different types of estrogenic foods are and assume if the word is associated with estrogen in any way, you must avoid it. This cannot be further from the truth.[19]

In fact, adding approximately 40mg of phyto-estrogens, including non-GMO soy and flax seeds daily is very protective and recommended.[20] Xeno-estrogens are phthalates from plastics. Conventional hormone replacements, non-organic meats, and herbicides and pesticides all throw off our hormone system, and they are also called endocrine disruptors and can lead to *abnormal cell proliferation and growth* – exactly what we **do not want** in cancer!

FOODS THAT IMPROVE GUT HEALTH

Since most of our immune system is located

in our gut, it only makes sense to feed our gut the correct nutrients to ensure that the environment, or microbiome, is balanced. Fermented foods, such as sauerkraut, miso, and kimchi all contribute to a healthy and balanced gut flora. These foods go through a process called lacto-fermentation where natural bacteria feeds on the sugar and starch in the food to create lactic acid. During this process, enzymes, probiotics, omega fatty acids, and B-vitamins are all created, along with preserving the food into a more digestible form. The end result is the reason why increasing fermented foods is fantastic for your digestive system, and these foods should be eaten daily. The true definition of fermentation is "the chemical breakdown of a substance by bacteria, yeasts, or other micro-organisms, typically involving effervescence and the giving off of heat."[21] It's common to see foods like milk, soy, and vegetables (cabbage, carrots, turnip, beet root, and green beans) fermented in order to preserve them longer and make the nutrients more absorbable. These fermented foods should all be added to your daily diet for optimal gut health.

ALKALIZE YOUR BODY THROUGH FOOD

What does it mean to alkalize your body? Your kidneys determine whether food turns into acid or alkaline once transferred to your blood. When looking at pH levels, we want to know which foods turn acid or alkaline in the body, and surprising to many is that this is not necessarily related to which foods happen to be acidic or not. With the help of our lungs and kidneys, our body is amazing at regulating the exact balance of acidity and alkalinity. The gist of it is that for us to be functioning optimally we want our body to be more alkaline than acidic. A normal blood pH level is 7.40 on a scale of 0 to 14, where 0 is the most acidic and 14 is the most alkaline. When it comes to food, most fruits and vegetables promote alkalinity, since their final breakdown product is bicarbonate (alkaline), whereas eggs, animal proteins, and dairy all increase sulfuric acid, resulting in our body becoming more acidic. We want to increase the foods that are alkaline forming or are full of potassium and magnesium.[22] The only accurate way to test your pH is through a blood sample, but urine and saliva are easier samples to extract for assessment so are most commonly done.

The pH of food cannot be determined by how your stomach reacts to it. For example, things that give off more acid from your stomach creating heartburn do not always mean the end result in your body and blood will be equivalent to more acidity. For example: let's consider lemons and citrus fruits. Lemons, limes and other citrus fruit have a pH level of 2, meaning that they are very acidic fruits and because of this high acidity, your body may be aggravated and experience heartburn symptoms after ingesting them. However when fully metabolized in the body, the pH of these fruits becomes a 7, meaning its end product is alkaline and not acidic and very healthy for us.

One fact that many people are not aware of is that cancerous tumors create their own microenvironment. Abnormal cells will use sugar for energy and create lactic acid as a byproduct.[23] It is in fact the abnormal cells creating this acidic environment without any outside influences. Knowing this, it makes our food choices that much more important. If eating a diet rich in acidic foods like grains and animal proteins, you are only adding fuel to the fire.

Your goal is to create your diet to be the opposite of what cancer feels comfortable in, a diet rich in fruits and vegetables, promoting alkalinity, with the added benefit of them being rich in vitamins and minerals. This will be sure to make the cancer cells uncomfortable within your body and will prohibit their growth.

Homework– Being aware about making adjustments to your diet each day.

1. Add foods into your diet daily that act as proteasome inhibitors, as they increase the breast cancer resistance protein BCRP. Try to add apples, onions, grapes, cabbage, broccoli, and organic green tea to your daily routine.[24]

2. With the exception and minimal amounts of organic red wine, avoid alcohol altogether. According to research, strong evidence shows that alcohol drastically increases breast cancer risk by 30-50% in premenopausal and postmenopausal women.[25] Many women express that alcohol helps them relax at the end of each night. If you feel you must have

a glass of wine, it NEEDS to be organic, free of pesticides, and herbicides, and at maximum one ounce a night. I realize that this is not a lot. So learn to sip– and add some deep breaths for additional relaxation benefits.

3. Increase foods that are breast cancer protective, like beans and lentils. Try to transition to ninety percent plant-based foods with a large variety of colorful fruits and vegetables.

4. If eating animal products, they must also be organic; free from pesticides, herbicides, hormones and drugs. They must also be grass-fed. Remember with meat consumption, you process and absorb everything that the animal eats and has come in contact with.

5. Choose low glycemic index and glycemic load foods. This is especially important for low active or overweight people or people who have been on hormone replacement therapy.

6. Include fresh organic vegetable juices. It is the best way to keep up with your body's nutritional demand. Juicing vegetables, such as celery, carrots, kale, and beets are very helpful.

Recipes will be included in the "recipe" section of this book.

7. Eliminate grapefruits from your diet. Even one fourth of a grapefruit will inhibit the estrogen clearing cytochrome P450 cyp3A4 enzyme in the liver.[26,27] This is enough to increase risk of breast cancer by as much as 30%.[28]

8. Include healthy fats with each meal. For example unheated olive oil, avocado, coconut oils, nuts and seeds are great additions.

Step 5: Fasting Protocols

In a book about enhancing nutrition, it seems odd to have a whole chapter dedicated to how you can live longer by not eating. However, this is the truth, and thousands of studies back the benefits of fasting. Before going into the research, let's go back in history, back to the primitive days, when we did not snack all day long, and instead spent most of our days being active, and sometimes only consuming one meal a day. Food was looked at as a means of survival, not for "entertainment" purposes or something to do out of "boredom".

Today, our mindset of diet and eating has changed because our culture has changed. For example, we say that we must all have breakfast, to "break the fast," and eat small bites every two hours, and have three complete meals a day, especially when sick. When suffering from a cold or flu, we are told to eat more, to "keep up our energy". On the contrary, this could not be further from the truth.

When animals in the wild are sick, they rest and have no desire to eat until their bodies heal and they build their strength back up in time. Humans are the same way – when we are sick, all of our energy must go into our vital organs for survival. Do not be mistaken, energy is needed for your body to heal properly, but when forcing food into your ill system, this energy should not be going towards the breakdown and metabolization of these foods. According to Hipprocates, the forefather of medicine, fasting enables the body to heal itself. Fasting means you are restricting calories for a minimum of twenty four hours, and depending on desired results, can last up to several weeks.

According to a review by Dr. Longo and Dr. Fontana of the University of Southern California, restricting calories without depriving critical nutrients, is the most potent and reproducible physiological intervention for increasing lifespan and protecting against cancer in mammals. Fasting reduces the levels of a number of anabolic hormones, growth factors and inflammatory cytokines, reduces oxidative stress and cell proliferation, enhances autophagy (cell destruction) and several DNA repair processes.[1]

EATING IS WASTING USEFUL ENERGY

By limiting the times when we eat our energy can be conserved and be focused on detoxifying and cleaning up waste products that have been stored in our bodies for years and years. Several studies show prolonged fasting during the sleep phase (called intermittent fasting) will positively influence carcinogenesis and metabolic processes that are associated with risk and prognosis of breast cancer.[2] Intermittent fasting (IF) is much less intimidating. It is a complete avoidance of calorie intake for thirteen to eighteen hours daily or alternating a fasting day with a normal intake day. The studies supporting (IF) show that 36% of breast cancer remission rates are increased by simply introducing a thirteen-hour fast per night.[3] It's incredible to know that according to the science, refraining from eating from six p.m. until seven a.m., gives you so much power in your own body's ability to help extend your life and this does not seem like that difficult of a task.

One reason is fasting this length for this amount of time can support how your body regulates sugars, as well as supporting enhanced sleep quality.

Both are important in the face of immune strength and cancer fighting abilities. Another main reason why fasting is so important is due to a process called "autophagy". Autophagy means your body is cleaning itself up. The longer you stay away from food, the more effective your body can go through this process. There is no herb or drug more effective at cleaning up old waste than what your body can be trained to do naturally.

Now, what exactly does it mean to avoid food? Does that mean drinks too? The answer is not simple – it depends on you. Every time you eat something, your pancreas releases insulin to help get the sugar/carbohydrate into your cells. The underlying reason why fasting is so effective is because you are limiting how often your body produces this insulin spike. So, every time you have a meal, a piece of fruit, vegetables, or even one peanut, insulin is being released from your pancreas.[4] Think of your daily routine: you wake up in the morning, have a wholesome breakfast, and then within that hour, you find yourself sipping a cup of tea with milk, and then another hour later you have some carrots or fruit, then lunch and another snack, dinner, another snack, and maybe before bed you have another cup of warm tea to relax. This is potentially sixteen hours of food constantly going into your system and a constant stream of insulin spikes. We know that insulin is a powerful growth factor for cancer cells, so understandably, these spikes will help provide your cancer cells with a protective shield, and your goal is to break this shield down.[5]

BREAKING BAD HABITS

This pattern of constant eating is the exact habit we need to break and get away from the mindset that we need food to be constantly entering our body in order to survive and thrive...We don't!

One sign that you know you are completely dependent on food is that you get what is called *hypoglycemic* between meals. This can be recognized as being agitated, anxious, lightheaded, shaky, and what they call *"hangry"* when food is not in sight. The deeper reason this happens is because we need to improve how our body sees food in the first place. If you cannot wait for your next meal and are constantly thinking about getting food, what you will be eating next etc. I'm sure you are looking at the whole practice of fasting as an impossible feat.

The good news, however, is that there is a lot we can do to improve this process and it starts with taking baby steps. You need to start slow. If for years you were used to going from ten p.m. until six a.m. without food, extend that each week by an extra hour. Additionally, anything that contains sugar in it will spike your insulin levels, so have that coffee black, and only water during fasting times. Yes, even green tea or herbal teas may disrupt your fasting period. As described in the ketogenic section, there is only one way to know for sure what does and does not spike your insulin levels, and that's getting access to a blood sugar monitor.

You can purchase a glucometer online or at any local pharmacy if you do not have access to one already. To fully understand your insulin production, you would measure your blood sugar first thing in the morning, drink that cup of green tea, then half an hour later measure your blood sugar again. If you see no change, then, yes, you could continue to have that tea within your fasting period. If you see any change (up to 0.02 difference) then you know you need to stay away, and this includes all other teas as well.

If you are having a tough time regulating your cravings, and find yourself to be hungry all the time, I want you to realistically look at your relationship with food. Is it really hunger? Or maybe it is boredom? Or a social decision that reinforces more meals and calories than necessary? I personally have this issue in my own life. Every time I feed my kids I feel I need to try their food, or if I'm passing through my kitchen I'll grab a handful of nuts, or even an apple. Am I hungry and needing those calories to survive? Absolutely not! By constantly introducing foods, your body starts to rely on the excess carbohydrates and sugar intake, and it is less likely to produce energy on its own through ketosis.

Ideally we want to train our body to not rely on food for energy. One way to do this is cut out the snacks. Just having three meals per day will provide all the calories you need in a day. Each meal can be up to ninety minutes long, to ensure you have the time to get enough in. It's the habits we have created our entire lives that reinforce these eating habits.

Recognizing and acknowledging that these life habits are part of the problem will help you integrate the solutions.

A lot of us get confused with what it means to be hungry, and dopamine plays a big role in this. This is the neurotransmitter that allows us to feel happy and give us that "get up and go" state of mind. Food can be looked at just like any other addiction, such as drugs and alcohol. We reach for food, just like a drug, to help us feel better. Comfort foods are a way to self-medicate and give us a chemical our brain is missing. The irony here is that we always feel worse. When looking to feel better, we never choose broccoli or sauerkraut; instead, we want food high in carbohydrate, and this is the vicious cycle starting again – sugar high, sugar dip, then the cravings. Recognizing this pattern will help us curb the cravings. When you have a healthy insulin response, healthy gut, and are given the proper nutrients, you should not feel hunger. Our microbiome is amazing. In a healthy gut, it is responsible for producing dopamine and our happy-hormone, serotonin.[6] If our gut environment is off, we search for things to give us those outside feelings of happiness. Fasting and implementing fasting regimens will put the power back in your hands, and keep you from looking elsewhere for that dopamine feeling.

FASTING CONTRAINDICATIONS

Who should avoid extended fasts? If you are underweight and cachexic, this is not the time to fast. In that case, you can still do twelve to fourteen-hour fasts, but you will want to make sure that the ten to twelve hours you eat are filled with high caloric foods in an easily digested form. Also, you should not do extended fasts while pregnant. Pregnancy is not the time to do any restricted diets. In the case of type 1 diabetes, where the body is not able to produce its own insulin, this will require more attention given by a knowledgeable health care provider to individualize a plan to ensure sugar levels are not dipping too low. Despite these contraindicated cases for extended fasts, do not neglect the idea completely. Anyone can start with fasting intermittently and continue to watch sugar intake and control.

The whole premise of intermittent fasting is

not to control calories. You are still eating the same amounts; however, you are just eating less frequently and in a timed manner. Ideally, you will get a high volume of nutrient-dense calories from 11:00a.m. to 7:00p.m. But let's be honest, the foods we tend to gravitate to after 7:00p.m. are likely not the most nutritious snacks. So therefore by not allowing yourself to eat after 7:00p.m., you will automatically be cutting out those unhealthy food choices. Giving your body a break, and fasting each night (or day) is beneficial for energy levels, hormone balancing, brain health, immune regulation, and like discussed, detoxification.

Should *You* Fast?

After being diagnosed with breast cancer, you can assume that your body needs additional support and healing. In order to maximize how your body heals, make sure there is no additional waste in your body to take care of. This will allow the body to use its energies and efforts to heal from the abnormal cell growth. Taking part in a fasting protocol encourages your body to return to its natural state of health. By allowing your digestive tract to rest, your body can go into repair mode, and leaky gut can also be resolved. Any irritation to the lining of your colon from stress, drugs, herbicides, pesticides, overeating, sugar, alcohol, or processed foods, has the chance to repair. While fasting, insulin receptors are also able to become more sensitive, meaning you will become more effective at absorbing nutrients, leading to less symptoms brought on by hypoglycemia like being lethargic.[7] It does take some training, but with time, you will find that it is much easier to follow this regime. Long story short, if you want to do everything possible to get healthier and live longer, fasting is non-negotiable for you.

Fasting's Secret Weapon – Ketone Bodies

As discussed previously, we use ketones as energy sources, which are much cleaner and efficient than using glucose or sugar for energy. If you are constantly putting sugar or carbohydrates into your system, your body will never be given the chance to create these ketones.

As previously mentioned in Chapter 3 Step 4, the Ketogenic Diets section, there is a way to test whether or not you are creating ketones after a prolonged fast in the same way as a blood sugar finger prick. A ketone monitor, available from the American site Ketomojo.com will allow you to measure your ketone levels. But more specifically, it's the glucose ketone index (GKI) we want to know more about. You can only reach an optimal GKI if your blood sugar levels are low enough, and your ketone levels are high enough. For example, even if you have been fasting for long periods, your body may be under stress, and the liver when under stress will start to produce glucose, preventing your body from going into ketosis. So longer fasts, especially when stress is involved, make it even more imperative we have our levels checked regularly. All the effort of testing, and adjusting routines regularly is worth the overall outcomes of prolonging life, strengthening your immune system, and boosting your body's ability to heal overall.

Homework for proper introductions from intermittent fasting to extended fasts:

Intermittent fasting (IF) is a great way to start your fasting journey. Below are the steps to prepare your body to go from IF to extended fasting times. Remember, just like you wouldn't go from being a couch potato, to running a full marathon, training for a fast is the same thing. Stay in each step as long as it takes, feel comfortable, and do not move on until you feel ready.

Week one: Lengthen the time between dinner and breakfast to allow for a longer overnight fast, with the goal of thirteen or more hours, for example: be finished dinner by 6:00pm and do not eat again until breakfast at 7:00am.

Week two: Prepare your body to go into a longer fasting time frame, only eat three meals a day, with no snacks. Remember, do not limit how much you eat within these times, taking up to ninety minutes per meal.

Week three: Introduce one twenty-four hour fasting day (a.k.a. eat one meal per day) this week. You should only drink water and eat foods that do not spike your sugar levels (you need to test this to know what you can consume).

Week four: Start working with a healthcare provider to help you determine how often and how long to engage in a fast. One to three days will drastically help regenerate the immune system, and increase cellular protection against oxidative stress.[8]

Important note: If you are currently undergoing chemotherapy, water fasting two to three days prior to treatment and up to one day following treatment can optimize the efficacy of treatment and reduce treatment-related side effects.[9, 10, 11] However, only under the supervision of a qualified practitioner should this be a consideration.

Step 6: How to Feel Stronger through Detoxification

According to the Center for Disease Control and Prevention, there are on average 212 various toxins present in people's blood and urine.[1,2] These chemicals put a burden on our digestive, nervous, circulatory, and lymphatic systems. If you have a colon full of feces, those toxins are then re-absorbed and directed back to the liver, also called "autointoxication," and this process invites our system to experience a whole new level of toxicity. When your body is full of toxicity and not eliminated efficiently, it can no longer give energy for a strong immune system, and sets the stage for chronic diseases, premature aging, and premature death. There was a study completed with Dr. Frank Falct at Hartford Hospital in Connecticut to understand how the body stores chemicals and pesticide residues in breast tissue. This study specifically looks at the organochlorine class of chemicals, including DDE, which is an end product of the pesticide DDT, and PCBs. This was a case-controlled study which showed significant differences of higher levels in women with cancer versus those who had biopsies and did not have cancer.[3]

TOXICITY

Many chemicals in plastics, pesticides, herbicides, or flame retardants, are hormone mimics or hormone disruptors. Another dramatic correlation was the finding that when only three pesticides were removed from the food production line in Israel, there was a drop in over thirty percent in the age-specific breast cancer mortality rate in an entire decade. This is overly impressive, considering that for twenty-five years prior, the rates for breast cancer were on a steady incline.[4] These studies make the correlation of chemical related toxicity and breast cancer seem overly simplistic, having chemical residues in your body does not automatically predict cancer but the correlation is something we can not just ignore.

We all know the world we live in is toxic; and these chemicals are known carcinogens and they have estrogenic effects especially after years of our bodies absorbing this toxicity. Today it is time to give your body a break. At least once a year, a thorough detoxification plan must be done in order to properly detoxify our bodies. Proper detoxification is a very different approach than fasting. The foundations of an effective detoxification plan is done primarily through nutrient-rich foods and enhancing all your organs of elimination – **the colon, liver, skin, lungs and kidneys** – these are known as our *five organs of elimination.*[5]

OUR BODIES HEALING POWERS

When our skin suffers from an abrasion it is amazing how our body just knows what to do in order to heal itself. It is constantly repairing and building new cells in our system to ensure we stay healthy and safe. People don't need drugs to assist in what our bodies are born to do naturally. When we focus on strengthening our system, our bodies ability to just know what to do in order to be healthy is quite incredible. One thing many people do not know about their bodies is that they are constantly in a cycle of detoxification. When I mention the word 'detox', all I mean is that the body is cleaning and clearing itself of toxins. Like clearing out a clogged sink. We want all the excess food, cooking oils and sludge cleared out to ensure the piping is running strong, clear and clean, and while we are on the cleaning house analogy, consider also the replacement of your air filters, and while you are at it, updating and renewing the whole home. Once you start, you shouldn't stop at the first problem that you encounter, you should look at the whole home... just as I would and have encouraged you to investigate your entire body.

We have five main detoxification organs – the colon, liver, skin, lungs and kidneys. Every day, these organs support how our body gets rid of waste and I want to break down the job of each one to make sure you are doing everything possible to have them work their best.

THE COLON

"Healing begins in the gut." – Hippocrates

The colon is the captain of all the detoxification organs so it is important to start here. If the colon is backed up, all the other systems are also backed up. Even when we eliminate stool every day, there can still be common issues.

Considering the anatomy and structure of the colon and also how it's shaped, it can be challenging for garbage to be completely eliminated, as there are many small pockets where particles can cling to or become stuck. My first two years of clinical practice I also worked as a Colon Hydrotherapist and during those years I saw some pretty crazy stuff. Pieces of food, parasites, yeast overgrowth, things that should never be sitting and settled in anyone for long periods of time. Even patients who had regular daily bowel movements, would release unchewed food and things the patients said they hadn't eaten in years. One example was a cherry pit, after having not eaten cherries in years. This proves that even if you have a movement daily, it doesn't mean your body is eliminating waste consistently.

Drinking enough water is a huge part of softening stool and being able to eliminate waste daily. Ideally, every person should have a bowel movement at least eighteen hours after every meal; therefore, if you have three meals a day, you should have three bowel movements, accordingly. When we feel bloated and gassy, that means our colon microbiome is off and is not breaking down food properly. Instead, the food that is being consumed is just sitting there, fermenting, and leading to further toxicity.

Colon hydrotherapy is an excellent way to get rid of waste that has been sitting in the colon for years. At my clinic, Inside Health, colon hydrotherapy is a large part of the journey to health. Our colon is made up of several pockets called diverticula. It is very common and easy for food particles to get stuck within these pockets. The colon hydrotherapy treatment helps alleviate the waste from your colon, and we can also add other healing supplements to the treatment like, bentonite clay which further pulls candida (yeast) as well as parasites from the body. The addition of peppermint oil calms and soothes irritable bowels, and the addition of chlorophyll pumps up healing and nourishment. Chlorophyll and bentonite act as a weak binding agent, which helps to pull out toxicity and unwanted waste from the body. These methods are by far the most effective way to clean up our colon and in turn helps to detoxify the body.[6]

We are so used to the idea of drinking coffee, that the thought of inserting it anywhere else likely seems insane, but this method has been used for years. The use of organic coffee can be added to your colon hydrotherapy treatment to promote healthy muscle contractions within the colon, called peristalsis, which are needed to create healthy bowel movements. That's right, inserting coffee up your rectum is in fact very beneficial for healthy bowel movements.

One reason why coffee is excellent when added to the colonic, is because it also supports how our liver detoxifies. Coffee opens up common bile ducts and supports toxicity to be released from the liver, the gallbladder, and helps pull toxicity from the colon. Organic coffee can also be added to colon hydrotherapy sessions, or to enema bags to support how our liver produces glutathione, the most powerful antioxidant that we produce naturally.

It's best to take a chelating agent prior to a colonic or enema, such as a supplement called phosphatidylcholine (PC), or chlorella and then after a half hour, it will promote the removal of bile and toxicity elimination from the colon.[7]

The Benefits of Coffee Enemas [8, 9]

1. It stimulates the liver, our main organ of detoxification, to produce more bile. Bile is a bodily fluid that has a role in fat digestion and is able to dissolve fat soluble toxins for removal from the body through the gallbladder, small intestine, and colon.

2. It opens and relaxes the common bile duct muscles to produce a large flow of bile from the gallbladder into the small intestine. This allows the liver to rid itself of many toxins quickly and make it available to process more blood-transported toxins from the rest of the body. It encourages a systemic detoxification effect and greater overall state of well-being.

*All the blood in your body passes through the liver approx. every three minutes.

3. It supports the dilation of blood vessels through the effects of the coffee's theophylline and theobromine, further increasing blood flow to

152

the liver.

4. It increases glutathione s-transferase (GST) production, a key detoxification enzyme, by 600 to 700%, through the action of coffee's palmitic acid. GST shuttles toxins for binding with glutathione, which neutralizes them and carries them out of the body in the bile.

5. Last but not least, it speeds up the transit time of waste through our main elimination organ, the colon.

What you will need to perform a coffee enema at home:

- ❑ One enema kit – can be purchased online or through Inside Health Clinic
- ❑ Measuring cup
- ❑ Tablespoon
- ❑ Strainer
- ❑ Organic Coffee

How to make organic coffee to prepare for your coffee enema at home:

- ❑ Pour four cups of water using a measuring cup

into a pot. Place the pot on the stove.

- ☐ Bring the four cups of water to a boil. Once the water starts to boil, turn the stove off.

- ☐ Immediately add two tablespoons of organic coffee into the pot of boiled water and briefly stir the coffee. Then let the coffee and water sit for twenty minutes uncovered to cool.

- ☐ After twenty minutes, strain (and throw out) any coffee grinds, and allow coffee to cool completely until liquid coffee is room temperature.

Steps to perform the coffee enema at home:

1. Take out the enema tube/bag from its plastic envelope.

2. Add 500mL of the cooled down coffee into the top of the bag - then clamp the tube by pressing on the white lock in the middle of the tube.

3. After all air is removed from the tubing, hang the bag filled with coffee above your shoulder height, near your toilet.

4. Prepare the area with a pillow for your head and have a towel to lie on for comfort. You should

position yourself on your left side.

5. After lubricating the tip of the tubing with coconut oil or olive oil, insert the tip of the tube approx 1.5 inches into your rectum.

6. Open the white clamp, so the water can flow through slowly.

   • You can use the clamp or squeeze the hose with your fingers to regulate the amount of fluid. If you feel uncomfortable with the pressure building in your colon, close the hose clamp or squeeze the hose shut with your fingers to allow the pressure to subside. Then begin again at a slower inflow rate. Only put as much fluid in as your colon will comfortably hold.

7. Once the enema coffee is in your colon, gently remove the tip of the nozzle and tube and let it hang into a clean container, and start your timer for 15 minutes. Roll onto your right side and relax. Several minutes after being on your right side, you can rest on your back and then towards the end of your 15 minutes, roll onto your left side again.

8. Once you have held the coffee inside your rectum for 15 minutes, proceed to the toilet and release the enema. Stay on the toilet as long as necessary to allow a complete evacuation. A toilet stool that raises your knees toward your chest can be helpful, as can momentarily standing up and sitting down again. Do not push or clench in anyway to achieve evacuation. Relax your muscles instead.

How often do I need to incorporate coffee enemas into my routine?

Coffee enemas are ideally done as maintenance three times a week, although if necessary, they can be done daily as well. When your system is overly toxic, we can support the elimination of wastes through this fifteen-minute treatment. When you're ill, these treatments can be done every few hours to encourage quick elimination and a mega boost to your liver, supporting glutathione production to fight off unwanted organisms within the body. You can take additional agents that support healthy daily movements, such as magnesium citrate (this pulls water into your colon to soften stool), while rhubarb, cascara, and senna are more aggressive laxatives to get stool moving. Fiber helps to bulk up the colon and also promotes gut movement and the best choice of fiber is those that come from fruits, vegetables, and legumes. Incorporating psyllium hulls, flax, hemp, and all seeds on a daily basis will also naturally support daily bowel movements.

THE LIVER

Your liver is a dense, football sized organ that sits just beneath your lowest rib, on the right side of your abdomen. It performs approximately five hundred functions within our body. Glutathione is a powerful antioxidant that is produced in the liver, contributing to its main role in our bodies immune defense. Your liver filters your blood, removes harmful bacteria, viruses, toxins, and yeast. The liver is also your main fat burning organ and is in charge of hormone regulation. Despite how you may be feeling clinically, conventional testing may not always show a dysfunction or impairment in its function.

In Chinese medicine,   when the liver is

overwhelmed, a person develops a condition called *liver qi stagnation.* This is a common condition and symptoms present themselves as irritability, cramps before or during your period, low energy and difficulty sleeping, dark circles under the eyes, a yellow-coated tongue, a bitter taste in the mouth, headaches, arthritis, and the inability to digest fats.[10] To stress the importance of our liver, human beings cannot survive more than twenty four hours without a functioning liver. The next time you feel irritable and agitated, especially before your period, take note of the following instructions, because it's your liver that needs the extra attention. There are two phases to how your liver detoxifies. Phase one is where enzymes act like soap bubbles and it starts to break down (clean away) toxins into another form. Some of these toxins are ready to leave the body after phase 1 and others need to go through this phase twice. In phase two, these compounds are moved along one of six detoxification pathways, bound to a specific molecule, and escorted out of the body through our kidneys or colon. This process is called *conjugation.* The most important pathway is the glutathione conjugation pathway, which is needed to detoxify and break down carcinogens. High exposure to toxicity can exhaust our bodies reserves of glutathione, possibly increasing susceptibility to cancer.[11]

Another thing that can deplete our levels of glutathione is excessive exercise as well as alcohol consumption. Too much of either can block glutathione production, and will increase oxidative stress on the body, leading to an increase in free radical production and inflammation in the body. It is important that phase one and two of liver detoxification is supported, if it were to slow down, it sets up a perfect habitat for toxic build up.

Things that you should be aware of to prevent phase one from *slowing down* (a.k.a. having a "sluggish liver") are the following: Stay away from grapefruit, turmeric, and capsicum. Capsicum is found in hot peppers, cloves, drugs containing benzodiazepine such as antidepressants and valium, anti-histamines, ketoconazole (used in anti-fungal medications).[12]

Another issue that can arise is if phase one of your liver detoxification is sped up. Toxic compounds can be created from this faster process and can actually be more toxic than the original toxin that your liver is trying to cleanse. Some of the things that speed up phase one liver detoxification include some of the following: Known carcinogens; pesticides, paint fumes, and cigarette smoke.

Medications like phenobarbital, steroids, and sulfonamide, charbroiled meats, high protein diets, alcohol, toxins from intestinal bacteria, when in the blood stream all stimulate phase one of liver detoxification. This is only an issue if phase two cannot keep up with the speed of phase one.[13]

If you plan on taking on a liver detoxification protocol, it is critical you have as least one bowel movement a day, since a backed up colon can also create more stress on your liver, causing toxicity to be recirculated within. When the colon and liver are backed up, we can also start to get skin irritations like acne, resulting in toxicity expressed through skin. Each one of our detoxification organs rely on each other to function optimally.

One excellent way to support liver detoxification is to place castor oil packs over the liver area with heat.[14, 15] Castor oil is the oil made from castor beans, and when being made it is important the extraction method is free from a chemical called hexane. Hexane-free castor oil is available online and in most health food stores for purchase.

Castor Oil Pack Instructions

1. Cut at least four pieces of cotton flannel into approximately six inch by six inch squares.

2. Completely soak the cotton flannel with the castrol oil within a small clean/dry container.

3. The oil soaked cotton flannel is now your castor oil pack and is ready to use.

4. Place the castor oil pack (one piece soaked through but not dripping cotton flannel) on the upper right side of your abdomen, just beneath your rib cage.

5. Place a small clean cloth over the castor oil pack before applying heat.

6. Apply a heating pad on top, and leave it for about forty-five minutes.

7. You can reuse this castor oil pack approximately thirty times.

8. Cover and refrigerate after each use.

Applying castor oil packs at least three times a week can help to decrease stagnation in the body; accelerate blood and lymphatic movement from the liver, aiding in how this organ detoxifies your body.

Foods that detoxify the liver:[16]

- Flaxseed oil
- Fresh fruits and vegetables
- Garlic
- Onions
- Sesame seed oil, walnut oil, wheat germ oil
- Wheat germ
- Cold water fish
- Cabbage and other cole crops (i.e. mustard family)

Top nutritional supplements

- Black currant seed oil
- Evening primrose oil
- N-Acetyl-cysteine
- Milk thistle (Silymarin)
- Vitamin C (ascorbic acid)

- Coenzyme Q10

THE SKIN

Our skin is our largest detoxification organ. Through each of our pores, we are constantly ridding our systems of unwanted waste by constantly perspiring. Many of us try to block this process by wearing antiperspirant deodorant; however, this creates more toxicity in our system as we are applying unnatural materials to our skin in order to prevent it from completing a very natural and necessary task. Raising our bodies temperature purposefully regulates our metabolism and creates a sweat response which helps kill off bacteria and viral activity in the body that shouldn't be there. It is beneficial to sweat each and every day, whether it's by regular daily exercise and movement, through steam, or infrared saunas. Aim for a good sweat at minimum forty minutes per session at least three times a week.

To further understand the importance of sweating, consider when you have a fever; your body raises your temperature and creates a fever to kill off the bugs. We are taught from an early age to take a pill to reduce a fever and that a fever is harmful; however, a fever is actually our smart body detoxifying and doing what it knows best. In the same way, encouraging sweating is critical every day to prevent toxicity buildup.

The Ozone Sauna

The use of ozone therapy within a sauna session is an incredible way to drive impurities out of the skin. The steam from the sauna opens your pores, and ozone is then able to enter your body to eliminate things like metals such as lead and mercury. Likewise, this is the best way to get rid of skin infections like candida and eczema. At my clinic, Inside Health, we offer ozone sauna sessions that support immune systems with modulating effects which are beneficial towards fighting any abnormal cells in your body. Soaking in an epsom salt bath for thirty minutes will provide your body with additional magnesium and sulfur to support detoxification and correct those deficiencies.

Dry Skin Brushing

Toxicity can gather beneath the skin's surface from such common influences such as improper pH levels in body soaps, skin creams, antiperspirants, as well as any synthetic fibers worn next to the skin. Any of these items can contribute to a variety of skin problems and conditions.

When you do dry skin brushing you help your lymph system to clean itself of the toxins that collect in the lymph glands. You use a simple technique to improve the surface circulation on the skin and keep the pores of the skin open. This encourages your body's discharge of metabolic waste, resulting in an improved ability to combat bacteria as well as helping your skin to appear and feel healthier and more resilient.

Daily skin brushing is a technique using circular motions and pressure with a dry brush to stimulate circulation and support the elimination of dead cells, because we are constantly shedding dead, old skin and producing new. You can purchase organic bamboo brushes online, from amazon, or within the Inside Health clinic.

There are many benefits of dry skin brushing. It helps to tighten skin, helps digestion, removes cellulite, stimulates circulation, increases cell renewal, cleanses the lymphatic system, removes dead skin layers, strengthens immune system, improves exchange between cells, and stimulates your glands, thus helping all of the body systems to perform at peak efficiency.

How to properly dry brush your skin:

1. Buy a natural (not synthetic) bristle brush as it does not scratch the surface of your skin.

2. Buy a brush with a long handle so that you're able to get to areas of your body that are not easily reached when doing your own skin brushing.

3. Skin brush before showering or bathing at least once per day - twice for even better results.

4. Do NOT wet your skin - it will not have the same effect because this stretches your skin.

5. Do lighter strokes over and around your breasts, but do not brush the nipple and know your sensitive areas. Brush lighter in sensitive areas.

6. Brush each part of your body several times vigorously, and make sure to brush your entire body.

7. Start with your feet and work your way upwards.

Brush the soles of your feet first because they have nerve endings that will affect your whole body. Next, brush your ankles, calves and thighs. Then, brush across your stomach and your buttocks. Lastly brush your hands and your arms.

8. Always use brush strokes and circular motion towards the heart.

9. After brushing, take a warm bath or shower, followed by a cool rinse at the end to invigorate blood circulation and stimulate surface warmth.

10. Wash your dry brush every few weeks in water and allow to dry completely before your next use.

THE LUNGS

On a daily basis, we inhale air pollution, second hand smoke, smog, chemicals and gases. Many of us don't realize natural decongestants in the air that cause allergies such as pollen and the dust that surfaces on table tops in our homes are constantly being inhaled by our lungs and none are naturally supposed to be there.

Besides inhaling foreign objects on a daily basis, another problem that occurs with our lungs is our inability to breathe properly. Instead we breathe too quickly or too short. We should practice taking deeper breaths as a lifestyle habit change, as the best way to detoxify our lungs is through deeper breathing. Maximizing our breath will improve the oxygen and carbon dioxide conversion, which is a critical step to lung detoxification. Deep "yoga breaths" and diaphragmatic breathing *(put a hand on your chest and belly, deeply breathe in and feel the abdomen expand, while your chest stays still and on the exhale, breathe out, while feeling your belly button get closer to your spine)* also help.

Top lung detoxifiers include: N-Acetyl Cysteine (NAC), and glutathione, especially in the nebulized form, which means it is inhaled in a mist directly into the lungs.[17, 18] When breathing these in, you will notice that your lungs may produce mucus to help carry out the waste. When we're sick, that's exactly what we want – to spit out mucus and phlegm. This is our bodies' intelligent way to eliminate and detoxify. When we take a cough suppressant, this medicine suppresses what our body should and will do naturally.

Remember, we want that garbage out! So when you are feeling ill and your chest is congested, the key focus is to pull the toxins out. So breathe deep and spit up any phlegm that loosens through this process. A warm compress and a homemade menthol rub on your chest will also loosen the phlegm that is holding firm in your lungs and will provide some relief.

Natural Chest Decongestant Recipe [19]

   -1/2 cup olive oil

   -1 cup cold pressed coconut oil

   -30 drops mint essential oil

   -15 drops lavender essential oil

   -15 drops rosemary essential oil

   -35 drops eucalyptus essential oil

THE KIDNEYS

Your kidneys are a bean-shaped organ about the size of your fist. They constantly filtrate blood and toxicity, and excrete excess water and waste products in the form of urine. Each kidney contains seventy miles of filtering tube called nephrons and its function is to conserve water, glucose, regulate electrolytes, and to eliminate acid by-products from protein metabolism and other waste from the blood.

To encourage kidney function, the easiest step for you to do is drink more water. You need approximately half to a full ounce of water for every pound you weigh. With excess sweating, your water intake should be closer to the one ounce per pound each day. For example, if you weigh 150 pounds, you would drink 75 to 150 ounces of pure, clean water daily. Reverse osmosis and remineralized water is the best.

It is important to look at your source of water when you drink, ensuring that no lead, fluorine, and other chemicals are found in it. Filtered water is best to ensure these contaminants are removed; however, too much filtration can also create a mineral imbalance within your water, so replacing these minerals are key.

Underactive kidneys affect the bowel, lungs, skin, lymph, heart, blood pressure, nerves, and many other organs and tissues by increasing the levels of harmful acids in the bloodstream and by altering your electrolyte balance. The most dangerous waste products are generated by the breakdown of proteins. The kidneys, like the bowel, are very important organs of elimination.

Foods that support kidney function:[20]

- Watermelon
- Watermelon seed milk
- Pomegranates
- Apples
- Lecithin
- Liquid chlorophyll
- Parsley
- Raw juices
- Green leafy vegetables
- Asparagus

Drinks that support kidney function:

- Celery juice (It is high in organic sodium and keeps calcium in the body which helps prevent kidney stones from forming.)
- Pomegranate juice (It helps maintain the correct

pH balance in the kidneys to assist the kidneys in fighting infections.)

- Parsley juice
- Black currant juice
- Beet juice
- Asparagus juice
- Grape juices (Each of the above juices mentioned help promote the healthy functioning of the kidneys overall.)
- Goat Whey (It is another drink that is excellent for the kidneys, as it is one of the highest sources of organic sodium. It is also a good source of chlorine and calcium.)

Vitamins that support kidney function:

- Vitamin A, Vitamin B-complex, Vitamin C, and Vitamin E

Minerals that support kidney function:

- Calcium, Potassium, Manganese, Magnesium, Silicon, Iron, Zinc, and Chlorine.

Herbs that support kidney function:

- Juniper berries, Uva ursi, Parsley, Goldenseal, Slippery elm, Dandelion, Marshmallow, Ginger

THE LYMPHATIC SYSTEM

Although this entire lymphatic system is not a "detoxification organ" it is still one of the most important mechanisms for how our body collects and dispels waste. Our lymphatic system, unlike our heart and cardiovascular system, does not have a pump that helps to keep fluid in motion. Instead, the lymphatic system relies on our own movement of our bodies to help with movement. For optimal function, the fluid within this network of lymph needs to move. To do so, you can use a machine called 'The Vibration Platform' or 'Vibe Plates'. Inside Health uses 'The Pettibon System', a vibration platform, which is a whole body unit that improves lymphatic circulation. Using these units for five to ten minutes daily is recommended, and specifically prior to a colon hydrotherapy session to drastically improve results of elimination. Going for a twenty minute walk, making sure to swing your arms will also stimulate lymph flow. Taking contrasting showers is also an incredible way to boost lymphatic circulation. This means you would take your regular shower using your preferred warm temperature, but near the end of your shower, turn the water to as cold as possible for 30 seconds and then alternate back to hot for 30 seconds. Repeat this cycle three times, ending with cold water for best results. As annoying as this process may seem, your lymphatic and immune system will thank you for it and you will feel refreshed and more awake afterwards! Rebounding and trampoline jumping are an excellent way to move lymph also, with the added benefit of it being low impact on your joints.

List of recommendations for moving lymph fluid

- Rebounding
- Deep breathing
- Practice yoga for increased lymphatic circulation
- Regular exercise
- Increase your water intake
- Take care of your skin; what goes on your skin is absorbed into your lymphatic system, so switch to using natural and organic moisturizers and beauty products

Lymphatic drainage massage

- Contrast showers
- Going braless, so your breasts can move; make sure your bra is never too tight and avoid underwires (your bra should not leave red marks when you remove it)

MENTAL DETOX

A mental detox, or rest, is an important part of the detoxification process as all of our energy needs to go towards cleansing our bodies. High stress and worry induce the sympathetic nervous system and blood flow goes to survival mode. Our body detoxifies best when it is in the parasympathetic mode and has the ability to relax.

To encourage this state of mind, turn off your phones, practice breathing exercises, take warm relaxing baths, and do your best to remove mental stress from all avenues. Create healthy boundaries by understanding who and what in your life makes you feel overwhelmed and stressed and take a break away from them. If that means taking a leave from work to focus on your health, that is a sacrifice worth making to better your whole self.

Going to bed early is also key. The routine of getting a full night's rest, going to bed early, and getting up early is the way our body functions best. We are naturally in this parasympathetic phase during rest, so this is when our body works hardest to clean itself up and dispose of waste and toxins.

Do you notice that when you're feeling low energy, your body needs a rest? It's telling you something, so listen to your body and rest. Instead, most people feel like they have to keep going, grab a coffee, or reach for other stimulants, and push through this feeling instead of breathing and taking that much needed nap our body is yearning for in order to repair.

Homework for creating a healthy mindset:

- Set your timer for ten minutes each day to focus on your breath, calming your mind. Getting your body into a parasympathetic state takes practice.
  1. *Sit in a relaxed position, with your back straight and eyes focused on any object ahead of you.*

2. *As you breath in through your nose slowly; sense your breath. Fill your lungs completely, and then empty as you exhale slowly.*

3. *Without any thoughts interfering, count each breath starting from 1, 2, 3, and so on.*

4. *Keep breathing and try practicing this counting up to 100 without your mind being interrupted by thoughts.*

- At first expect this to be a challenge, but each day will get easier. Practicing your breath in a peaceful state of mind will start to become a habit.

Healing Crisis

When you are sick and going through a detoxification process, depending on how aggressive you are cleaning up, you will likely experience a "healing crisis". When cleaning up the body, it is normal to feel worse at first. Believe it or not, this is actually a good sign. The body is experiencing the same symptoms temporarily as it returns to the uphill road, eliminating toxic waste as it goes. This process is what your body needs to do to truly heal.

Once you have started the detox process, the odd headache, sore throat, tired feeling, bone ache, chill, or pain may appear, and this is all normal. When done properly, an organ in your body usually takes one to six months to detoxify and rebuild itself back to the point where it will function optimally again. However, depending on the severity of the condition, the organ(s) may require one month for every year that the problem existed. Chronic conditions may take longer than a year to truly heal, and those who are patient and persevere to the end are the ones who see results. Of course, this isn't to say that you won't gradually feel improvement, but to get to a point of "remission", you must be patient and let the body work at its own pace, not expect an immediate cure.

The healing crisis only occurs when the body is cleansed naturally, with correct nutrition and supplementation. The body has the strength and vitality to stand the accelerated healing process (therefore, there is no need to be anxious) and the body will take care of itself without any outside assistance (such as Aspirin and Tylenol, as these medications will only interrupt the healing process). The healing process can start within three days, or take up to three months when chronically ill, and it can last from one day up to twenty-eight days.[21] By eating correctly, the body may eliminate waste little by little at a time or may never experience a healing crisis at all. During a guided detoxification plan, it is imperative that we go at a pace that is right for you, based on your medical and disease history. Below is an example of what a seven day detoxification plan would look like, which optimizes all the five elimination organs.

SEVEN DAY DETOX PLAN

When your body is overwhelmed and your immune system is in need of a recharge, the best thing you can do to it is to detoxify. Clearing the body of bacteria, phlegm, mucus, parasites and years of toxicity needs to be done in this step by step process. It is important you are medically supervised or have the approval from your health care practitioner if you plan to take on the seven day detox plan below. If one of our elimination organs is congested or clogged, it will affect the rest. The daily regimen listed below is the basic supplement guideline to support detoxification, and supply your body with all the required nutrients it needs each day for optimal function. Even though calories are very minimal, you will likely be supplied more high quality nutrients in this one week than you would in a typical diet. Additional therapies such as colon hydrotherapy, coffee enemas, dry skin brushes, lymphatic drainage, and rebounding throughout each day is highly recommended and should be added to this program. They will all stimulate circulation, help clear congestion, and minimize a healing crisis that may occur throughout the week.

Day 1 to Day 5- The liquid cleanse
Product details are listed below

Morning

8:00am: 250ml of warm water + 2 capsules of *Clean Digestive

8:45am: *Detox Drinks 1 & 2* (Recipes can be found in the Appendix)

10:30am: 250mL of Organic Greens Juice (Recipe can be found in the Appendix)

11:00am: 3 *Capsules Clean Greens

11:30am: 250ml of *Herbal Teas

Noon

12:00pm: *Detox Drinks 1 & 2* (Recipes can be found in the Appendix)

1:00pm: Organic Greens Juice (Recipe can be found in the Appendix) + 3 Capsules of *Clean Digestive

1:30pm: Filtered Water plus Teas

3:00pm: 500ml of *Clean Greens Juice (Recipe can be found in the Appendix)

Evening

4:00pm: *Detox Drinks 1 & 2* (Recipes can be found in the Appendix)

4:30pm: 250ml Teas + 250mL Filtered Water.

5:00pm: 500mL Organic Soup (Recipes can be found in the Appendix) + 3 Capsules Clean Digestive

5-8pm: Teas + Filtered Water

Bed Time: 2 capsules Probiotics, Clean Bowels (if needed), 2 capsules High EPA Fish Oil

During this five day plan, add coffee enemas every morning, and colon hydrotherapy every evening. Regularly emptying the colon will ensure toxicity is not re-circulating throughout your body, this is the ultimate way to clean out your system. Cleaning on the deepest cellular level, the quality of stool coming out of your colon on day one will be drastically different than what is eliminated on day five, making the entire process very exciting!

Day 6 to 7 Transitioning from Cleanse to Solids

Coming off the liquid cleanse is just as important as the cleanse itself. During the detox plan, digestion slows down, and because of these changes, food must be introduced slowly.

Morning

8:00am: You should start your day off with a bowel movement. An enema or colon hydrotherapy can assist in this as well as help clean out remaining waste.

8:30am: *Detox Drink 1* + **plus one scoop amino acid powder** and *Detox Drink 2*

10:30am: 500ml of Organic Greens Juice and 3 *Capsules Clean Greens + **plus 1 probiotic**

11:30am: 250ml of *Herbal Teas

Lunch

12:00pm: 1 cup of vegetable soup (Recipes can be found in the Appendix) + **plus 2 Clean Digestive capsules**

Dinner

6:00pm: Lightly steamed vegetables and/or vegetable mineral broth, and /or vegetable soups + plus one small piece of protein (fish, organic tofu) + **plus 2 Clean Digestive capsules.**

OR Fresh Vegetable salad with baked tofu and tempeh + **plus 2 Clean Digestive capsules** (Recipes can be found in the Appendix)

Bedtime: 1 Probiotic (1 capsule *Clean bowels – If needed for regular / daily bowel movement)

During a whole body detoxification regimen, it can be even more challenging mentally than it is physically. It is important to rest and get to bed early each night. The week must be during a time where you limit commitments, more importantly to avoid the social pressures of eating. The first 2 days will be the toughest to get through. Many feel withdrawals, headaches, and fatigue, but once day three comes around energy starts to pick back up, and the entire process becomes more familiar. You will be shocked to feel energy throughout this program, when for years you have felt energy output was directly correlated to food input. Your body is amazing. Giving it the opportunity to take a break and truly heal will provide the exact healing powers your body needs to live longer and stronger in the face of any disease process, especially breast cancer.

What is in each supplement?

*Clean Greens:

Chlorella

Spirulina

Alfalfa leaf

Rose Hips

Red Beet Root

Broccoli Powder

Spinach Powder

Iodine from Kelp

*Clean Fiber:

Psyllium husks

Psyllium seed powder

Potassium bicarbonate

Burdock

Apple pectin

Flax seed

Marshmallow root

Ginger root

Slippery elm bark

Fennel seed

*Clean Bowels:

Magnesium oxide

Aloe vera

Senna

Rhubarb root powder

Prune powder

*Clean Digestive:

Amylase

Protease

Glucoamylase

Lipase

DPPIV

Papain

Bromelain

Marshmallow Root

Ginger Root

Apple Cider Vinegar:

Raw

organic

unfiltered (contains mother)

Liver Tea:

Silybum marianum folia

Taraxacum officinalis

Urtica dioica folia

Cynara scolymus

Galium aparine

Achillea millefolium

Kidneys/Blood Cleansing Tea:

Trifolium pratense

Galium aparine

Avena sativa

Medicago sativa

Urtica dioica folia

Smilax officinalis

Scrophularia nodosa

Probiotics:

Broad spectrum

High EPA Fish Oils:

EPA

DHA

Mineral Salts

Olive Oil:

Since every cell in your body is surrounded by a fat layer, fats are a critical component to your overall health.

• CHAPTER 4 •

Testing

Your body is constantly evolving, and now that you have a cleaner system to work with, it is important to understand where your body is on a deeper level so you can take the appropriate measure to make it stronger. In the medical field, blood, urine, and imaging are performed as routine checkups and measurements. However, there are many more options out there that allow us to see what's actually the root cause that explain the reasons *why* things happen in your body. The goal is to have as much information as possible and to know what happens in our body in ways we would never know, unless through another scientific lens.

Let's start with blood work. This list may be different than what your family doctor or oncologist will look at, but remember, we want to know the why, so we can fix and strengthen the body, not just attain an end result. I will include blood work that may or may not be checked by your family doctor or oncologist along with the names of the tests, why they are important, and how to achieve "optimal level," rather than the wide reference range that is typically given to tell you that you're "within a normal range".

BLOOD TESTING: *What we test and what we look for.*

<u>HA1c, fasting glucose and fasting insulin levels</u>

Understanding how your body processes sugar and its relationship to insulin.

HA1c <5%

fasting glucose <100mg/dL

fasting insulin < 25 mIU/L

<u>IGF-1</u>

A growth factor that is directly linked to promoting cell growth and proliferation. IGF level <92.7 ng/mL

<u>TSH, freeT3, freeT4, TPO, Tg, including antibodies</u>

Metabolic testing for thyroid health, including hypothyroidism and autoimmune conditions of the thyroid. If these levels are off, have your iodine levels assessed. Poor gut health, side effects of medications, and stress can all contribute to thyroid levels being off.

TSH <2.

Antibodies <30

Vitamin D

Vitamin D is a critical vitamin for cell differentiation, immune and hormone regulation.

Vitamin D 200-250ng/mL

CRP and ESR

CRP and ESR are typically inflammation markers and you want these levels to be as low as possible.

CRP <3, ESR < 5.

Liver and Kidney enzymes

Liver and kidney enzymes: see fluctuations based on various medications or stressors on the body, including cancer.

ALT/AST <40 units/L

Ferritin and Iron

Ferritin is another measurement for inflammation. Cancer cells love iron and use it to stimulate cell division/proliferation. Ferritin levels are optimal between 35-75.

G6PD

This is an important test to have, prior to any high dose Vitamin C IV therapy is performed. High dosage is considered to be over 20,000mg through intravenous. If you are missing this G6PD enzyme, your healthy cells cannot tolerate that high load of vitamin C and will cause cells to blow up (hemolysis).

CBC

CBC stands for: complete blood count. This test gives us an overall picture and indicator of what your red blood cells, white blood cells, and neutrophils look like. Typically, when any of these levels are too low, certain conventional and integrative cancer therapies cannot be performed and can be dangerous.

TESTING FOOD INTOLERANCES

There are a few ways that you can measure which foods cause more inflammation in your body, and one test is through muscle testing. This is a hands-on approach to test what foods weaken your body, and which ones strengthen your body and which have no impact at all. If you think we are all beings living with different energies, you know that everything has a frequency to it, including our foods, our bodies, our clothing fabrics, emotions, furniture, and the list goes on. When we are faced with certain objects or think certain ways, that in turn creates messages that are then passed through our bodies.

For example, during an EEG test (brain imaging), the monitor picks up on various impulses and measures brain activity such as alertness, excitement, and drowsiness. In the same way, when heart monitoring, an electrocardiogram will pick up electrical charges that travel through the heart. Thinking a certain way and being around certain people as well as eating certain foods can affect this signaling pattern. When muscle testing for foods, the basic premise is that our body is constantly picking up on frequencies, and those frequencies are telling our immune, nervous system, and cardiovascular system how to act.

In another example, when we come into

contact with someone who is negative or angry, our brain releases chemicals called neurotransmitters that immediately sends our body into distress, making our heart uncontrollably race, and we go into a sympathetic response. Additionally, if we have a presentation or test coming up, those high stress and anxious thoughts will affect our body, giving signals of restlessness or even the urge to have diarrhea.

Another source of these neurotransmitters are also released from our gut, aka your *second brain*. The plexus of nerves located in the gut are called the *enteric nervous system*, explaining why there is a powerful gut-brain connection. The foods we put into our body will affect the health of the cells in our gut, affecting this nervous system, and from a cellular level drastically affecting how our body reacts to various situations.

IgG testing is another way to test for food sensitivities.[1] These are the foods that will trigger an immune reaction and lead to inflammation in your body. A finger prick sample of your blood is taken to the lab and tested against over a hundred different foods to see which ones spark an immune reaction called IgG. Our goal is to get rid of all foods that trigger this pro-inflammatory response, because overtime, eating the wrong foods has been linked to several chronic conditions, such as low energy, digestive disorders, weight issues, and arthritis. Many people know which foods they are allergic to, but it's rare that they know of their food sensitivities. Food allergies are the ones that trigger our body to produce massive amounts of a chemical called histamine, which leads to anaphylaxis. This fatal condition causes the throat and esophagus to inflame, swell, and cut off air to our lungs. This reaction can also cause hives, rashes, and other non-life-threatening reactions. In scientific terms, this type of reaction is called a type-I hypersensitivity reaction, caused by the degranulation of mast cells, or basophils, that is mediated by immunoglobulin E (IgE).

The measurement of food intolerances is different, and this testing will show which foods cause an inflammatory reaction, even up to seven days later, making it difficult to detect on our own. Now, you may think, "This is a cancer book; I want to know which foods specifically are linked to my cancer growth." Since each one of us are so different, the specific foods that come back as positive on your food sensitivity testing will be the exact foods that you need to avoid to prevent inflammation and the growth of cancer. Bringing down daily inflammatory triggers from food is an imperative step to living longer and fighting cancer more effectively.

When food intolerance testing is done through a lab, there are also drawbacks as well; if you eat the same foods all the time, they may all pop up, meaning that they are starting to irritate your immune system. If you have a leaky gut, almost all foods (or over twenty of them) will seem like they are negatively affecting your body – even foods like broccoli. If on your report, you see more than twenty foods tested positive, this is an indication that you need to look deeper into your digestive tract, suspecting a weakness there like "leaky gut". If the integrity of your gut is not strong, foods will be able to leak into your bloodstream creating an abnormal immune reaction, which could be the reason that healthy foods like broccoli and lemons appear on the test results, leading to more inflammation.

Prior to testing, for most accurate results, you want to make sure you include a wide variety of foods into your diet for at least 72 hours prior. This includes all grains, vegetables, fruits, meats, dairy and spices. If you do not have certain foods in your system prior to testing, there is no way your immune system can elicit a response and they may show up as false negatives on the report. Also make note that any medication that affects your immune system, like steroids and antihistamines will affect reliability of the results also. Therefore if you are going to spend money on this testing method, eat a wide variety of foods, and try and avoid these medications for at least three days before giving your blood sample.[2]

TESTING HORMONE AND STRESS THROUGH URINE

Even if your breast cancer is not estrogen or progesterone positive, having your hormones evaluated is a critical step to fighting any cancer and living stronger. Estrogen is a hormone that promotes cell growth, testing how your body metabolizes and breaks down this hormone is extremely valuable. You also want to know how estrogen is being methylated. If your body is not methylated well, it can be a major source of damage to your DNA and can be contributing to turning on other cancers. Equally important, this testing can determine hormone metabolites like 2-, 4- and 16- hydroxyestrone. Through this test you can understand how your body deals with exogenous estrogens, from foods, drugs, and environmental sources.

We know that if estrogen is not broken down into certain forms, it negatively affects our DNA and can stimulate abnormal cell growth. Hormone testing, especially for breast cancer, will show you what your adrenal glands and stress response looks like. If you have high stress, and are constantly producing cortisol from your adrenal glands, this will lower immune function, weakening your ability to fight abnormal cells in the body. Most women that have come to visit the clinic show their cortisol levels are in overdrive and on the verge of burnout. Having this test performed allows us to intervene at certain points throughout the day to control this cortisol release that plays a role on not only sex hormones, but how we deal with life each day. This also measures our oxidative stress, another measurement to see how much stress the body is affected by on a cellular level.

Testing hormones through blood is not as clinically relevant, considering it measures the amount of hormones that are floating around your bloodstream, and not necessarily what is being absorbed by your tissues and being used. At our clinic, Inside Health, we can measure the available amount of hormones your body is able to absorb and then use, but only through urinary metabolite testing can this be accomplished. The preferred test kit is called DUTCH Complete.[3] It is a comprehensive urinary assessment of adrenal and sex hormones and their metabolite levels throughout a twenty four hour period. It also includes other valuable measurements such as organic acids, melatonin, and levels of oxidative stress within the body. This comprehensive report allows an individualized treatment plan to be put into place, furthermore optimizing your cancer fighting plan.[4]

TESTING YOUR POOP

By now, you know that the health of your gut needs to be at the forefront of your cancer fighting plan. By looking at your poop, we can point out the obvious. Pieces of undigested food implies poor enzyme reactions and if your poop floats this indicates poor fat metabolism. The only way to truly know what is going on in your body, on a deeper level, is to have your stool fibers tested. This includes testing for anything harmful living in your gut. Such as microbes, bacteria, parasites, yeast, and fungus. Without any obvious symptoms, infections may have been living in your digestive tract for years. Since most of our immune system is located in our gut, we can also check our IgA immune response, which will affect the way your immune system fights microbes and anything pathogenic within it. Anything abnormal found in the gut, will distract how our immune system functions, and directly affect how our bodies fight cancer. The test kit used in the clinic is called the GI MAP and it uses quantitative polymerase chain reaction (qPCR) technology to detect parasites, fungi, helicobacter pylori (h.pylori), ebstein barr virus, and more. By targeting the specific DNA of each organism we can determine the smallest of abnormalities.[5] After the stool sample is sent off to the lab, results will allow us to prepare a treatment plan focused on optimizing gut function, which will drastically impact your overall health. The gut microbiome dictates the effects of diet, digestion, immune, metabolic and even neuroendocrine functions. Taking a deep look into your stool will help understand the root cause of any imbalance in your system, including breast cancer.

TESTING FOR METAL & NON-METAL CHEMICAL PROFILES

It is virtually impossible to avoid all sources of chemicals entering our body. Like noted in the detoxification chapter, we all have over 200 chemicals within us, passed down from our mothers at birth. Recent and long-term exposures of carcinogens can be found in your body, coming from various foods, herbicides, fungicides, pesticides, pollution, environmental toxins, plastics, xenoestrogens, household cleaners, shampoos, body cleansers, and makeup. Metal and non-metal chemical profiles can be objectively measured to assess the current level of accumulated toxins in your body. Toxicity occurs when the net retention exceeds what your body is able to tolerate, determined by the difference between rates of assimilation and excretion of these metals. Doctors Data provides test kits that measure levels of aluminum, antimony, arsenic, barium, beryllium, bismuth, cadmium, cesium, gadolinium, lead, mercury, nickel, palladium, platinum, tellurium, thallium, thorium, tin, tungsten, and uranium which are being stored in the body. These metals do not float around in our blood stream, and because of this the only way to accurately test for these toxins is through a urine test. This urine test should take place before and after taking a chelating agent. Strong chelating agents, such as EDTA, DMSA and DMPS, act like a magnet to these metals.[6, 7] The chelating agent is used in metal detoxification as well as sequestering hidden metals from deep tissue stores which are then mobilized to be excreted as urine from the kidneys. Testing before and after taking any of these agents helps to understand what you have been acutely exposed to, versus net bodily retention. When it comes to inflammation and how enzymes are being activated and how minerals are being absorbed, it is critical we understand how our body is able to eliminate these chemicals.

Lifestyle changes should be made based on these results, and understanding where these exposures may be coming from and finding alternatives is key to making these changes. For example, for tests showing high levels of lead, you want to consider getting your drinking water, and bathing water assessed, and purchasing filters to avoid intake of this metal. Mercury is another example. If you have dental fillings that are metal amalgams, it doesn't matter how much detoxing you do as levels will always test high on labs, because any heat in the mouth will create a mercury vapour, and off gassing from that amalgam starts in the mouth and travels through your systemic circulation. After eliminating the source of the metal or toxin, ongoing protocols that include liver detoxing and metal chelating agents are used to support their removal.[8, 9]

LIVE BLOOD ANALYSIS

Ever wonder what your blood looks like under a microscope? With the aid of advanced microscopic and video equipment, this fascinating assessment takes a finger prick of blood, magnifies it, and is able to give an immediate and live nutritional and cellular health assessment. This assessment is very different from conventional blood work, because when looking at live blood you can check your health on a deeper cellular level. You gain immediate insights towards your health, including indications for leaky gut, vitamin and mineral deficiencies, toxicities, liver stress, inflammation, microbes, parasites, tendencies toward allergic reaction, excess fat in your circulation, arteriosclerosis, and indications on how your immune system is being activated. It is very beneficial to have this test performed prior to starting any treatment plan, gaining insight to any areas that may be deficient. After a plan is put into place, blood analysis can show how the treatments have changed your health and show healing on a cellular level.

A TONGUE EXAM

An assessment of your tongue, looking at its colour, shape and coat, can give various insights to what is going on in your body. It is not a substitute for medical health assessments, it merely gives more information about how your body is functioning and its overall health.

Different areas of the tongue represent different organ systems: liver, spleen, heart, and kidney. All these organs must work together and be in balance for us to be strong and healthy, especially when fighting breast cancer. So what should your tongue look like? Its colour should be a light red, too light may indicate anemia, and too dark may suspect high stagnation or inflammation in the body. The tongue should be smooth, and not have any cracks, or not be puffy or swollen or have indents along the edges. Coating on the tongue should be thin and clear. A thick white coat may indicate excess yeast in the body, and a yellow coat could mean infection. Take note, or even better, take pictures of what your tongue looks like each morning, as your health changes, your tongue will change as well.[10]

IODINE TESTING

Iodine has been shown in literature to have several anti-cancer properties.[11] A simple way to test if you have sufficient iodine levels is to apply one drop of two percent iodine solution to your inner wrist which will leave a brown stain on your skin. If your body is deficient of iodine, the brown coloured stain will disappear within a few hours after your skin absorbs it. If you have sufficient amounts, that spot will still be there approximately twenty four hours later. Signs that you may be low in iodine include thyroid symptoms such as:

-Swelling in the neck

-Gradual or unexpected weight gain

-Low energy

-Hair loss

-Dry, flaky skin

-Feeling colder than usual

-Changes in heart rate

-Trouble learning and remembering

ZINC TALLY TESTS

Our immune system relies on various

minerals, including zinc, to become activated and strong.[12] To test for sufficiency, hold one teaspoon of liquid zinc in your mouth for fifteen seconds. If you do not taste anything right away, it may indicate a zinc deficiency. If you get an immediate perception of taste, you likely have adequate levels. Other signs that you may be deficient in this mineral include:

-Altered/loss of taste and smell

-Anorexia (lack or loss of appetite)

-Apathy

-Ataxic gait (uncoordinated movements)

-Decreased immunity

-Depression

-Diarrhea

-Excessive hair loss

GENETIC CANCER CARE & ONCOBLOT TESTING

Ongoing damage to genetic material and your specific tumor are both extremely unique to each individual. This random genetic instability can also play a role in the outcome of how various cancer treatments work on your specific type of breast cancer. Because each person has a unique genetic code, responses to various treatments vary greatly. One study found that a proportion of people who will respond to chemotherapy treatment varies from five to eight in every one hundred (Royal North Shore Hospital, 2005). Personalized testing should be considered to further understand your individual health on a genetic level. Personalized genetic testing can be ordered through a company called RGCC, to potentially identify certain forms of cancer, and also to monitor cancer's progression or response to ongoing cancer care.[13]

Blood work can be done which focuses on screening and analyzing cancer cells at its early stage. Typical mammograms can detect a mass once it reaches 4.5 trillion cells, whereas the oncoblot can detect a mass of only 2 million cells. . A sample of blood is drawn, to detect circulating tumor cells, which are cancer cells that have detached from the original tumour and circulate through your blood and lymph to potentially create a secondary tumour site. It specifically detects a protein called ENOX2 that exists only on the surface of cancer cells. It can be used for detecting cancer, as well as every 3-6 months to gauge how effective your current treatment plan is. Visit RGCC-group.com and Ivygenelabs.com for more details.[14]

OncotypeDX
BREAST RECURRENCE SCORE TEST

During a biopsy or lump removal there is important information you can gain from your tumor. If you have estrogen receptor positive, or HER2-negative breast cancer, the OncotypeDX Breast Recurrence Score test can help you decide on treatment options.

Here is the criteria sourced from oncotypeIQ.com:

For women older than 50 years of age:

- **Recurrence Score of 0-25:** The cancer has a low risk of recurrence. The benefits of chemotherapy likely will not outweigh the risks of side effects.

- **Recurrence Score of 26-100:** The cancer has a high risk of recurrence. The benefits of chemotherapy are likely to be greater than the risks of side effects.

For women age 50 and younger:

- **Recurrence Score of 0-15:** The cancer has a low risk of recurrence. The benefits of chemotherapy likely will not outweigh the risks of side effects.

- **Recurrence Score of 16-20:** The cancer has a low to medium risk of recurrence. The benefits of chemotherapy likely will not outweigh the risks of side effects.

- **Recurrence Score of 21-25:** The cancer has a medium risk of recurrence. The benefits of chemotherapy are likely to be greater than the risks of side effects.

- **Recurrence Score of 26-100:** The cancer has a high risk of recurrence. The benefits of chemotherapy are likely to be greater than the risks of side effects.

The Oncotype DX DCIS score analyzes the activity of 12 genes. You and your doctor can use the following ranges to interpret your results for DCIS:

- **Recurrence Score lower than 39:** The DCIS has a low risk of recurrence. The benefit of radiation therapy is likely to be small and will not outweigh the risks of side effects.

- **Recurrence Score between 39 and 54:** The DCIS has an intermediate risk of recurrence. It's unclear whether the benefits of radiation therapy outweigh the risks of side effects.

- **Recurrence Score greater than 54:** The DCIS has a high risk of recurrence, and the benefits of radiation therapy are likely to be greater than the risks of side effects.

There is so much power in knowing your body on a genetic and cellular level. Advanced testing and using the described tools to understand where your body and your cancer are gives a tremendous advantage to fighting your cancer more effectively. To stay on top of the ever-evolving changes that are going on in your body I recommend repeating blood tests and nutritional live blood analysis every three months, and a comprehensive stool test and urinary hormone test at a minimum of once a year. Your body has an amazing ability to heal, and when you take the guesswork out of it, you can have much more confidence in the treatment plans you integrate into your health by optimizing your cancer fighting journey.

• CHAPTER 5 •

Advanced Cancer Therapies

At this point, you have worked hard at improving all your detoxification organs and strengthened how your body and immune system works. Now it is time to learn about all the highly researched advanced therapies that can be considered after speaking to your integrative health care provider.

There are two main categories when it comes to fighting cancer cells. First, are the agents that act as a pro-oxidant (meaning the ones that have the ability to kill cancer cells directly). In the mainstream world of medicine, these include chemotherapy and radiation therapy. In the naturopathic world, they would include high dose vitamin C, high dose melatonin, artesunate, and oxygen therapies.

TOP PRO-OXIDANT THERAPIES
High Dose IV Vitamin C Therapy

When vitamin C is supplemented at low doses orally, for example; 1000-2000mg, it is considered an antioxidant, and this supports the clean up of free radical damage. What we want to do is deliver vitamin C at pro-oxidant levels, ranging from 50,000 to 70,000mg through an IV. This treatment provides oxidative effects and is selectively toxic to cancer cells. Within tumors, vitamin C generates a large amount of hydrogen peroxide, which is extremely lethal to cancer cells.

You might now be wondering, how can this high dose of vitamin C and hydrogen peroxide not affect healthy cells also? It doesn't, due to the fact that healthy cells produce an enzyme called catalase and cancer cells do not. Catalase directly neutralizes hydrogen peroxide so it cannot damage your healthy cells. Back in 1970, the Nobel Prize winning scientist, Dr. Linus Pauling, along with British cancer surgeon, Ewan Cameron, were the first to discover the benefits of high dose vitamin C treatments for terminal cancer patients. The studies through the years focused on high dose vitamin C taken orally. This route is not a cancer therapy. In clinics, there have been thousands of patients who optimize their cancer kill potential by participating in high dose IV vitamin C therapy three times a week, and with or without chemotherapy, and with spacing treatments out to once a week after the cancer is stable and in remission. IV vitamin C therapy can arrest growth and spread of tumours and has had an extremely high success rate with all types of breast cancer.[1]

High dose vitamin C therapy during chemotherapy acts as a supportive treatment and it will improve drug uptake while reducing drug induced resistance by supporting p-glycoprotein activity. P-glycoprotein is an important cell protein that regulates drugs within the cell. On the contrary, IVC treatments should be avoided during radiation, as it will increase pro-oxidant adverse effects. Testing for kidney function, specifically eGFR and creatinine levels are needed to ensure your body can handle this high dose of vitamin C. Also, we need to check for an enzyme called G6PD, because if missing, you are not a candidate for high dose IVC therapy. When your red blood cells do not make enough G6PD and you experience added stress on the body, your red blood cells can break apart, and this is called hemolysis, which will lead to anemia. Symptoms of low G6PD activity include dizziness, low energy, especially worse after exercise. Other than low kidney function, and low G6PD activity, there are no other contraindications to having this pro-oxidant therapy incorporated into your cancer plan.

Artesunate

Artesunate is one of my favourite herbs for breast cancer, due to the fact it is beneficial for so many conditions. It has been traditionally used for killing parasites, such as malaria, however in clinic it is most recognized for balancing hormones, reducing excess estrogen, and prolactin and having strong anti-cancer properties. Cancer cells are down-regulated from the use of artemisinin, and they are approximately one hundred times more susceptible to dying versus healthy cells.[2] Cancer cells have more transferrin receptors, making ferritin (stored iron) levels much higher. High ferritin is also another indication of high inflammation, a hallmark of cancer. Cancer cells use iron to grow and replicate faster, which is a reason to never supplement with iron, unless you are truly anemic.[3]

In cases of low iron, heme iron is the best

source, taken three times a day with meals after therapy is complete. Artesunate gravitates to these high iron fueled cells, and becomes activated to directly induce apoptosis a.k.a., cell death. Because healthy cells have the enzyme catalayse, It has a protective effect, and will not be damaged in the process.

Artesunate also disrupts blood supply to tumors, inhibiting angiogenesis. This herb is also fantastic at lessening inflammation. I have seen several patients whose CRP and ESR levels drastically reduce on blood work after implementing this protocol. It's important to note all antioxidant supplements like green tea extract (EGCG), grapeseed, oral vitamin C, glutathione, and vitamin E are to be avoided at least four hours before and after this therapy. Adding high dose vitamin C acts as a phenomenal synergy, which is why these two IVS are done back to back. Speak to your health care practitioner to carefully evaluate lab work and determine if this therapy is recommended for you.

OXYGEN THERAPIES

It is well known that the human body cannot

function without oxygen. Your body is made up of mostly water, and water is over 90% oxygen. We require this oxygen to generate chemical reactions, detoxify waste, and for each cell to function. Based on Otto Warburg's Nobel Prize research, all degenerative diseases, including breast cancer, are due to lack of oxygen within us.[4] Oxygen has two molecules of oxygen, and ozone has three molecules of oxygen. With that additional atom of oxygen, it is extremely powerful and can be used in medicine, which is called an oxidative therapy, or ozone therapy. If you are low in oxygen, due to a lack of exercise, poor diet, environmental pollution, high stress, improper breathing, or smoking, then your body is unable to sufficiently eliminate toxicity. Immune cells are more effective when they are well-oxygenated, and as with exercise, they are highly beneficial for the body. Using this super powered form of oxygen, at very specific concentrations, has the ability to kill viruses, yeast, parasites, and bacteria.[5]

Ozone and Breast Cancer

Once ozone enters the body it breaks down into oxygen species and oxidative molecules that become specifically toxic to cancer cells without harming your healthy cells. High oxygen within our tissues will improve healing and our immune response to infections. When a cell drops below 40% of normal oxygen levels, the cell energy production switches to a process called fermentation, which is an inferior method of energy production. In response to this low oxygen state our body reacts with an extreme intelligence and will find alternate survival sources to grow and replicate, such as growth factors like IGF.

Medical grade ozone is formed from pure oxygen, going through a generator with an electrical current to form ozone. Ozone (O3) is very unstable, it breaks apart very easily, so when injected into your body, the extra oxygen is quickly taken in and is beneficial to all healthy cells, yet destroys all the bad, because all pathogens, including cancer cells, dislike ozone.[6]

Ozone can be administered to any area of the body needing healing. For example, ozone can work administered vaginally to kill yeast during a yeast infection, rectally for infections within your digestive tract, such as diverticulitis, and colitis and inhaling the ozonide is also a treatment method. After being filtered through olive oil, it may treat infections such as bronchitis, and pneumonia. Ozone can be infused into a carrier oil and applied topically for any infection, including use for oral lesions developed from chemotherapy side effects.

My personal preference for oxygenating therapies is through blood. Approximately 200ml of blood is removed and saturated with ozone, creating oxygen rich blood, which is then added back into your bloodstream. There have been no negative side effects to this treatment. Although not everyone is a candidate for injectable ozone, patients who do undergo this therapy generally express feeling more energy, and less chemotherapy side effects. The benefits of this therapy also include a boost to one's immune system, increased superoxide dismutase, increased catalase, detoxifying the liver, and protective properties during chemo and radiation therapies.[7]

Ozone Sauna

There are many benefits to regular use of the ozone sauna and here is a list that goes far beyond just sweating:

1. Relaxes and loosens muscles by reducing the buildup of lactic acid and increasing muscle flexibility.
2. Oxidizes toxins so they can be eliminated through the skin, lungs, kidneys and colon.
3. Boosts blood circulation, helping injured muscles to repair quicker.
4. Stimulates vasodilation of peripheral blood vessels relieving pain and speeding the healing process.
5. Eliminates bacterial and viral infections of all kinds.

It is common during or after chemotherapy that your immune system is compromised and more prone to picking up infections. I have seen the body get over incredible skin conditions with the use of this sauna, including shingles, candida, eczema, and difficult to treat ulcerations.

Sweating is an important part to all detoxification protocols, and eliminating waste that has been in our body for years. Humid heat opens the pores which allows the ozone through the skin to the bloodstream where it can travel to the fat and lymph tissue. Drug or environmental toxicity typically stores itself in your body's fat cells, and ozone therapy helps assist in its removal.

During the treatment you are sitting on a towel and after approximately 20 minutes of sweating, it is typical to see a black streak form on the towel you have been sitting on. After laboratory testing, it is proven to be an accumulation of metals being excreted from your body! Metals serve no purpose, but can create a lot of inflammation in your body. Typically this process takes years for metals to be excreted by any other method. The combination of heat and ozone is a powerful tool to clean up your system, eliminate waste, and give your immune cells a boost to fight any abnormal cell, including cancer cells. For more information visit: www.ozonegenerator.com

MISTLETOE

Mistletoe is a semi-parasitic plant that comes in various forms: from apple, oak, pine, and elm trees. It has been used to strengthen your body's resistance, and boost immune function. Research on mistletoe, originating in Europe, have gained popularity and are widely studied in cancer therapy.[8, 9] This therapy is injected under the skin, or into an IV bag. In clinic, the patients who seem to be in remission longest have always had mistletoe as part of their cancer treatment plan; boosting immune function, keeping energy high, and keeping tumor markers low for years. For subcutaneous injections, it is healthy and normal for a small loonie sized red area to appear, showing a positive immune response. Any larger reaction may indicate an allergy and another type of mistletoe should be used. For example, Type P is the strongest, and most suited for post menopausal breast cancer, but if you react to a low dosage, switch to Type M. Type M is also very strong, however most indicated for pre-menopausal women. Type A is the type you use if you are going through chemotherapy and or radiation. You can switch based on where you are in therapy. Ideally this therapy is used in IVC vitamin bags, however can be used in pure saline also.

Mistletoe Self-Injections

Due to the fact injections may need to be done 1-3 times a week, many patients prefer to do these injections themselves at home. After being shown the technique, you will find it is easy to do yourself and very manageable from home.

1. Open the ampule by applying pressure to the red dot, and snap backwards.

2. Place the needle into the ampoule, and draw back the syringe.

3. Pinch area of abdomen with thumb and index finger, and inject needle just beneath the skin, at a 45 degree angle.

4. Dispose the needle into a sharps container that can be found at any local pharmacy.

You always start at the lowest dose and only increase after no red reaction appears. It is ideal to have a redness and swelling at the injection site, maximum 5cm in diameter. This is a cytokine reaction, and indicates your immune system is being activated, which is a very healthy sign. Any reaction that is larger than the stated above measurements like swelling in the face, itchy rash, or shortness of breath, may indicate allergy, and you need to stop using mistletoe immediately. First set of injections should always be done initially in the presence of your doctor, who can guide you on the type that is most suitable, and can monitor dosage progression and frequency of treatments.

MELATONIN

This hormone is produced in your pineal gland in your brain, initiated by the absence of light. There are numerous studies showing that shift workers, like nurses and factory workers are at higher risk of breast cancer due to suppressed melatonin production. The benefits of having adequate levels of this hormone could be written in a book completely on its own, but to list a few; this hormone directly inhibits cancers growth, modulates hormones, and makes tumors more hormone dependent leading to better treatment responses. It also improves how your body processes sugars and glucose, increases apoptosis, balances stress hormones and cortisol production, and improves chances of survival in terminal cancers.[10]

From studies, it shows melatonin levels tend to be lowest in estrogen positive cases of breast cancer. If you have troubles sleeping, or have had years of shift work, you can almost assume that you are low. The DUTCH urinary hormone testing checks for current levels that your body is producing, you want those levels to be on the high end of normal. You can increase your levels naturally by avoiding artificial lights (screen on television or cell phone) at night, creating a pitch-dark room while sleeping, and daily meditation or breathing exercises. Even without any sleep issues, of all the patients I have tested with cancer, they have all shown melatonin being on the low end of normal. So even if you feel that you sleep really well, this does not actually mean that your body is producing a healthy level of melatonin. Dosing for cancer is minimum 10mg each night. Over 10mg would be the dose needed to produce pro-oxidant effects in cancer, versus 2-5mg acting as an antioxidant and beneficial for jet lag and restoring sleep rhythms.[11]

TOP ANTIOXIDANTS

It is shocking to learn all the sources of free radical damage that we are exposed to. Cancer pro-oxidant therapies are the most obvious, however things like alcohol, pollutants, cigarettes, pesticides, fried foods, and even exercise all contribute to the amount of free radical levels within the body. You read that correctly, even exercise will increase aerobic metabolism and increase free radicals. The majority of cancer fighting agents, including chemotherapy and radiation, and the above pro-oxidant therapies all contribute to our bodies oxidation load. This is why antioxidants are indirectly a critical component to your anti-cancer plan. Antioxidants are also known as *free radical scavengers*, that help eliminate or neutralize damage caused by the aforementioned. They work by donating an electron to free radicals before they can damage other cell components. Therapy must be aimed at increasing the amount of antioxidants in our cells, especially in breast cancer.[12]

In short, antioxidants are not a cure for cancer, but they help manage the oxidative stress that is elevated throughout all cancer treatments. Below is a categorized list specific to breast cancer types. Your integrative health care provider will help determine which supplements are most beneficial to you. These supplements should also be avoided at the same time of doing chemotherapy or any oxidative therapy, since it will decrease its effectiveness. I typically recommend waiting until all chemotherapy and radiation is complete, however each case may be integrated into your plan differently.

Antioxidants plus hormone regulators

Breast cancers that are estrogen and/or progesterone positive will benefit from the below list.[13] Other indications that your hormones may be off are if you have a history of painful or irregular periods, cyclical mood swings, acne production, and conditions such as PCOS in the past or present, concluding that you may also benefit from the list below.

-EGCG (green tea) – 700mg three times a day.

-DIM or I-3-C – 200mg per day

-Sulforaphane from broccoli– 800mcg per day

-Grape Seed extract- 500mg two times a day.

-Iodine – 10mg daily

-Inositol – 4 grams daily. Increase to 8 grams daily if you also experience anxiety or symptoms of OCD.

Antioxidants plus blood sugar regulators

Patients whose blood work shows high IGF levels, high 12 hour fasting glucose, and high HA1c levels, should consider the products listed below, along with a low glycemic diet, as both will be beneficial.

-Berberine – 500mg 3 times a day with food.[14, 15]

-Modified Citrus Pectin–5 grams daily (Pre and post surgery take 5 grams three times a day for at least 6 weeks).[16, 17]

TRIPLE NEGATIVE BREAST CANCER

This type of breast cancer tends to be more aggressive and faster growing than other types, with higher chances of returning after initial diagnosis. Clinical protocols focus on the fact that this type of breast cancer has many active hormone receptors, including AR+ and can respond to anti-androgen therapies, such as the below supplements:

-Green tea (EGCG) – 1,000mg/day

-Indole-3-carbinol – 200mg/ day

-Curcumin – 600mg 3 times a day[18, 19]

-Co-enzyme Q10 –200mg[20, 21]

-Selenium – 40 mcg 2 times a day[22, 23]

-Grape seed extract – 500mg 2 times a day.

-Sulforaphane – 800 mcg daily

-Quercetin – 500mg 2 times daily[24, 25, 26]

MODIFIED CITRUS PECTIN

Derived from the peels of lemons, limes, oranges and grapefruit, modified citrus pectin (MCP) is another top multifunctional food based product that all breast cancer patients should take advantage of. When you are first diagnosed with a tumor, it can do little harm, until it starts to spread. If cancer cells cannot proliferate, it cannot metastasize to other parts of your body. The main action of MCP is to inhibit the overexpression of galectin-3 molecules in the body, controlling how cells divide, regulate, grow and spread.

Several studies support its use in cancer by directly stimulating immune system activity, and preventing abnormal cellular growth. Several immune markers are enhanced with MCP by significantly increasing T-cytotoxic cells and natural killer cells which all play a role in inducing programmed cell death and eliminating unwanted cancer cells. Removing heavy metals and ridding the body of candida is another protective role that MCP offers, making it an excellent product that has an overall clean up effect on the body [27, 28]

There is only one quality source that I prescribe which is PectaSol-C. This product excels in its purification process and is the only standardized source. I would not compromise on quality when investing in a product like this.

Supplementing with this product is essential prior to any lump or tumor removal. During a biopsy, There is a 50% risk of your cancer spreading from biopsy, and 1-2% risk post surgery through a process called tumor seeding.[29] Prior to any procedure is the most critical time to prepare, and take all precautions to prevent cancer spread. The daily dose would be anywhere between 6 - 30 grams every day (in divided doses). This is a non toxic product and its effectiveness is directly correlated with dosage.

ANTIBIOTICS

The thought of giving antibiotics goes against

everything I believe in as a Naturopath, however, there have been studies showing their effectiveness in eradicating breast cancer stem cells. Examples are azithromycin, doxycycline, tigecycline, pyrvinium pamoate, and chloramphenicol.[30] Remembering to supplement with broad spectrum probiotics between treatments will help protect yourself from gut dysbiosis.

MODULATE CANCER STEM CELLS

Stem cells have the ability to replace old, injured, mutated or toxic cells in your body. In order for cancer cells to grow at the accelerated rate that they do, they need to engage additional stem cells to encourage growth within the cancerous tumor. Chemotherapy and radiation may actually increase cancer stem cell growth, resulting in tumor cells moving freely through your body and capable of forming new tumor sites. It is critical you support how your body manages these stem cells. Top researched agents used to improve therapeutic response, and prevent cancer recurrence include:

-Curcumin

-Metformin (selectively inhibits cancer mesenchymal stem cells, and IGF-1)[31]

-Vitamin A[32]

-Vitamin C[33]

-Vitamin D3[34]

BERBERINE

Berberine displays powerful anti-cancer activity by inhibiting tumor formation and boosting immune function. It is an antimicrobial herb from the Oregon grape root, coupled with strong anti-inflammatory properties. Berberine has also been shown to inhibit the growth of candida albican, which is a common side effect of antibiotic usage. This herb is a must if you also have issues with blood sugar regulation, and your breast cancer is driven predominately by IGF-1. Studies show berberine will reduce insulin resistance, without causing blood sugar dips. Clinically, it has been shown that the reduction in insulin resistance and blood sugar control has an equivalent performance to the conventional diabetic drug Metformin. Many diabetics, and people with high IGF-1 levels on blood work can ask their health professional if this herb can be taken in replace of the medication Metformin. Its main mechanism in its power against cancer is it destroys free radicals, and is anti-mutagenic. Dosages would range between 300mg - 500mg two to three times daily, and taken with meals.

OPERATIVE & CONVENTIONAL CARE

For small tumours, under 1 cm in diameter, and for the most success you should have the lump removed right away. For premenopausal women, it is highly recommended that the timing of your surgery is done ideally about a week before your period starts. Studies show that when you are in the luteal phase of your cycle, there is less of a chance of blood vessel growth and cancer spreading, a process called angiogenesis. On the other hand, if your cancer has spread beyond the breast tissue, a mastectomy is not recommended, it will cause distant sites to grow faster, therefore surgeons generally recommend against breast removal at this time.

Make sure to avoid any natural ingredients that

may cause bleeding or clotting issues at least 72 hours before surgery. This includes the supplementation of garlic, curcumin, and green tea (EGCG), as well as no more than 3 grams of Vitamin C, ginseng, CoQ10, Vitamin K, and Omega 3 fish oils.

Pre-Surgery

Your focus when preparing for surgery is on building immune function and managing the potential for metastasis. The following supplements are recommended one week prior to surgery:

-Zinc – 60mg daily[35]

-Vitamin A – 10,000 IU 2x daily

-Protein powder (whey isolate) – 30 mg 2x/day[36]

One day before surgery:

-Modified citrus pectin – 4 capsules twice daily to prevent cancer from spreading post biopsy or surgery.

Specifically for scar reduction care:

-Rosehip oil[37]

-Superficial injection therapy to support breaking up scar tissue.

Post-Surgery

After surgery, your body will be in mode to recover. You will need extra support for wound healing as well as preventative care for potential metastasis. This care can continue for at least 2 months post surgery. Some of the following supplements are suggested:

-Modified citrus pectin – 4 capsules twice daily

-Green Tea/EGCG – 700mg three times a day[38]

-Vitamin E – 400 IU daily[39]

-Zinc – 30mg twice a day[40]

-Vitamin C –1,000mg 3 times a day[41]

-Probiotics – enteric coated, 2-3 capsules daily[42]

-Bromelain – 500mg 3 times a day[43]

-Fish Oil – 3 grams daily[44]

Chemoprotective

These supplements are to help protect you from chemo induced stress on your body. Supplementing starts on day one of chemotherapy treatment and carries through to day 30 post treatment.

-Melatonin – 20 mg at bedtime[45]

-Mistletoe Lectins – During chemotherapy, only

type A is suitable.[46]

-Astragalus – 1 tsp tincture daily[47]

-Reishi mushroom – 3 capsules twice daily[48]

-B12 – especially with neurotoxic drugs such as cyclophosphamide, taxanes, and platinum drugs.[49]

-Fasting – 24 hours pre, 48 hours post chemo.

Radioprotective

Avoid antioxidants, especially Vitamin E, manganese, iron and copper during this time. What you should supplement to help protect your body under radiation treatments are listed below:

-Melatonin – 20mg+[50]

-Omega fish oil – 4,000mg daily[51]

-Berberine –300mg 3 times a day[52]

-Organic red wine – 1 glass daily[53]

-Ginseng (eleutherococcus senticosus) – can also be used for low energy[54]

-Zinc – 30mg twice daily with food[55]

Supplements For All Types of Breast Cancer

-Vitamin D3 – 2,000 IU to 3,000 IU daily (strong hormone regulator and prevents cancer growth; careful in estrogen positive, high doses are estrogenic)

-EGCG from green tea– 700mg three times a day (95% polyphenol concentrate (low caffeine). It is impossible to drink the amount of tea needed to reach this amount (over several dozens of cups), and it stops cancerous cell growth)

-Vitamin E and Wheat Germ

(never in the d-alpha tocopherol form; highly protective; induces apoptosis)

DRUG INTERACTIONS AND SIDE EFFECTS

Common conventional drugs used to keep cancer in remission often have side effects such as joint pain, vaginal dryness, and hot flashes. After speaking to your healthcare provider, here are a few options that are safe and highly recommended that can help you replace deficiencies and combat these side effects.

Tamoxifen

Side effects include low energy, nausea, vomiting, chills, constipation, hot flashes and stomatitis.[56] To help combat these effects:

-High dose of Vitamin D (more than 2,000-3,000 IU) which can inhibit an enzyme that is capable of raising E2 estrogen.

-Soy isoflavones may decrease side effects of hot flashes

-Increased drug effectiveness with melatonin, indole-3-carbinol, acetyl-L-carnitine, CoQ10, quercetin, and Vitamin A, green tea extract/EGCG.

Herceptin

Herceptin contributes to an increase of five times more likely to experience heart disease, heart damage and/or heart failure.[57] It is mandatory to strengthen heart tissue throughout this therapy, including:

-Omega 3 fish oil – 2 grams daily

-Crataegus oxyacantha[58]

-Grapeseed extract

-Vitamin E

-Coenzyme Q10

Aromatase Inhibitors

These are a class of drugs that have side

effects of joint pain and carpal tunnel syndrome. The following list will help reduce these side effects:

-Omega 3 fish oils

-Vitamin D3 along with 120mcg of Vitamin K2.

-Devil's Claw Root extract[59]

-Melatonin

-Vitamin B6

Natural Aromatase Inhibitors

- Indole-3-carbinol (or DIM)

- Melatonin

-Quercetin

-Grape seed extract

-Reishi

-Red wine

-Resveratrol

-Flaxseed

-Zinc

-Natural progesterone

-Soy genistein

MULTI-DRUG RESISTANCE

With recurrent cycles of chemotherapy, and

various drugs, you may wonder why results are less effective as time goes on. Part of the reason is due to the fact that cancer cells can develop a condition called multi-drug resistance. There are natural agents that have the power to reverse this effect, including:

-Quercetin

-Green tea (EGCG)

-Ginseng

-Curcumin

-Melatonin

-Vitamin C

-Vitamin K3

-Ozone therapies

ACUPUNCTURE

As part of an integrated plan, acupuncture is a fabulous addition to reduce various side effects of chemotherapy, conventional drugs, or for health optimization. Specifically, in the clinic, this therapy excels when treating lymphoedema, hot flashes, joint pain, libido, energy, anxiety, sleep issues and well-being. For optimal results, this non-invasive therapy is side effect free, and should be used at least once a week.

PEMF THERAPY

Our health and disease fighting abilities are greatly determined by the state of health that our cells are in. Pulsed electromagnetic field (PEMF) therapy is a vital component for all breast cancer treatment protocols because its main purpose is to energize and restore cells to a normal balance. Science has proven that our bodies project their own magnetic field, and that all seventy trillion cells communicate through electrical frequencies. We know this is true when measuring heart rhythm and brain wave activity. All energy is electromagnetic in nature. All atoms, chemicals, and cells produce electromagnetic fields (EMFs). When this electromagnetic exchange stops, our body's function slows and begins to shut down.

Research has shown cancer cells function at a significantly lower electrical voltage than regular healthy cells. In order to slow the aging process, and reduce cellular dysfunction, re-energizing and rebalancing our cells is necessary.

A few of the benefits of using PEMF therapy

is that it gives a major energy boost to healthy cells. It supports detoxification while enhancing cellular metabolism and helps restore cells to a normal, healthy balanced electrical state. It also reduces pain, inflammation and accelerates wound and injury healing by helping the body grow new bone and nerve cells, while improving gene expression and restoring the body's energetic balance.

It is a phenomenal enhancement to IV Vitamin therapies, post colon hydrotherapy detoxification and as a standalone treatment to optimize each cell. In 1982, FDA first approved the use of PEMF therapy to improve the rate of healing broken bones. After thousands of studies, in 2011, the FDA approved this therapy in the treatment of cancer.[60]

The treatment involves lying flat on a mat, for eight to twelve minutes, ideally every day. It is safe, painless, and non-invasive. Most patients who use this therapy end up investing in one for their homes, to make it realistic to use every day.

SUMMARY

Advanced cancer therapies are widely used

among patients with breast cancer. There are many purposes to adding advanced therapies to your current plan, including preventing drug induced deficiencies, enhancing drug effects and outcomes, supporting healthy cells, and overall building your system. Your cancer journey is extremely unique, as you can see by all the categories, there are many variations to your personal plan. For ultimate success, there needs to be this integrative approach. It is highly recommended you have an open dialogue with your healthcare providers regarding these advanced therapies to know which ones are most beneficial to you. You deserve to feel strong throughout this entire process, and taking advantage of all therapies will enhance your cancer fighting success.

• CHAPTER 6 •

Obstacles to Healing

Now that you know what steps are needed to live longer, you have all the tools to strengthen your health and fight cancer more efficiently. It's very common to see people who have been stuck in a lifestyle that does not support health. Remember, these habits were mainly how you were raised and what was shown to you as being normal. Most people are afraid to step outside of that paradigm because that diet and lifestyle has served them for many years. A famous quote from Albert Einstein is, "The definition of insanity is doing the same thing over and over again but expecting different results". This is true, and we cannot live life out of fear of change. We need to ask ourselves what will happen if we don't change? You are risking your life by not changing and adopting a healthier lifestyle. But now is your chance.

But it's a lot of work!

I know what you're thinking: *"I know other*

people who have seen a naturopath, and it seems like a lot of work. Getting healthy and strong seems like too much effort; I've been so tired – I can't even imagine going through a program like this. I am too ill and too fatigued to cook and prepare meals. My life is too busy to follow such a routine. I don't have the time or energy to take care of myself, to cook and to be healthy, to find a support team, or to learn strategies and routines." I hear this a lot from first time patients, friends, and even family members that aren't eating healthy, making healthy lifestyle choices etc. that this shift in perspective, *"Is just too hard"*. But even still, your life literally depends on it. Most people see health as an overwhelming process, and that's because it's easy to fail when you don't have accountability for yourself and your future.

Accountability

You do have professional guidance that will keep you on track, and make sure you follow all the steps. Support team communities share fears and struggles and are made up of groups of breast cancer survivors, just like you. It's easy to feel alone in this journey but being a part of a larger support group will give you more strength throughout this process. There are several communities within the clinic Inside Health with like minded women all going through similar challenges. It's proven when you have people around you who are positive and encouraging you are more likely to succeed.

Too Expensive

You might think, "It's too expensive to get healthy", but what is your life worth? Your money means nothing if you're dead. People try to save their money or choose healthcare by price shopping, and that is the worst way to choose the person who is going to extend your life.

After a diagnosis and after doing everything your doctor says, the current medical model implies that you need to just wait until the next imaging and bloodwork to make decisions. However, we know that is not true. You can start now, by doing everything possible, putting the power in your hands and increasing the chances of improved results on your path to living longer.

I'm In Remission

Once you start getting some energy back, you

may start to become complacent, feeling like you can start returning to how your lifestyle was pre-cancer, and cancer will love that. Instead, creating the strongest body for your future will increase the likelihood of cancer staying away. Cancer specialists may also say that anything beyond chemo, radiation, and surgery is a waste of time and money, but we all know that mindset is simply outdated and archaic. Being told that you're *cured* or in *remission* is no reason to get too comfortable or complacent regarding your health. It may be tempting to slide into old health routines, but once your energy starts coming back, you'll be feeling so good, taking care of your health is now just an important staple in your life and cannot be seen any other way.

Being Powerful

With the many obstacles you can imagine, cancer has a life of its own, and is able to break through all of the obstacles that you create. Cancer is clever, but so are you. You have all the tools and everything inside of you to fight this disease, and create a body that cancer does not want to live in. I want to give you the opportunity to have your body,

and immune system function at its highest fighting
potential.

• CHAPTER 7 •

The Ultimate Guide

This book was written to give you hope, strength, and encouragement to fight smarter and more effectively in the face of breast cancer. I want you to take advantage of all the tools and resources that will make this journey to living a healthier and longer life successful. The more information and understanding you have regarding how your body works, the more sense your path to moving forward and setting yourself up for long-term remission will be. My ultimate wish is for you to feel strong, brave, and courageous. Up-leveling your strength and will to survive will be the biggest hurdle, but without that, it's challenging to truly get well. Your surrounding community and team will remind you why you've got this – you're fierce, and nothing can stop you!

I have seen miracles in the past decade while treating people with cancer. The power of the mind and body amazes me each and every day. You are unique, as is the way your cancer is presented, and

I am passionate to see you and your health journey reach the next level, by providing all the knowledge and support you need in this overwhelming field of cancer. I am excited to support your confidence in moving forward. A large part of this knowledge is understanding how your body works, because we are essentially treating your body, and when your body is stronger, it can always fight cancer more effectively. You now have the easy tools to apply to your daily life, which sets your body up for optimal function and health.

You now fully understand why cancer grows, and that's a huge part when fighting it effectively. Now that you have this reference guide and understand the lingo of how and why cancer grows, it makes sense why certain therapies work, and why certain ones do not. You can look back on your life and have an idea regarding why your cancer started in the first place and having this knowledge now gives you a drastic amount of power.

I hope you never look at food the same, instead looking at it as a fuel and choosing only high vibrational foods. Overhauling what goes into your body, specific to your cancer, will change you on the deepest cellular level, each day supporting the creation of a healthier version of yourself. By applying food, nutrition, and fasting principles, you are building a fierce cancer fighting army and equipping them with tools which will aid you immensely.

Not only have you learned how food can give you that critical foundation, but you've also learned how to clean your body on the deepest cellular level, and I am so excited to see you do so. By feeling recharged and clean and clearing out the years of garbage and toxicity that you have been holding onto, your body will finally have a chance to breathe, recharge, and tackle any disease process that comes its way. After you have cleaned up and improved how your body functions, the tests listed in this book are an incredible resource for you to understand where you stand. There is no other measurement to your current health status than getting those objective measures. We can use those results to elevate your health even further, creating treatment plans unique to you and helping you continually fight hard. Taking advantage of all the proven treatments and therapies will allow you to fight your cancer more effectively, and by knowing which ones are right for you, based on your personalized lab work, will ensure that you are utilizing all the tools to fight cancer more effectively. I want nothing more than for you to feel empowered. At this point, you should feel hopeful that you are able to tackle this fight more effectively. It is now time to take this step-by-step guide and put it into action, breaking through all the false beliefs regarding why you cannot break through those barriers to get well. The majority of this action plan can be done in the comfort of your own home; however, the more advanced testing and therapies need to be done through a clinic such as Inside Health and by a licensed naturopathic doctor who has all the expertise in the detox methods and cancer-specific therapies.

My wish for you is that you start implementing these steps into your daily life right away. Breast cancer is a wakeup call and the moment is now to change the quality of your life. Collectively integrating this plan into your life will offer so many more opportunities for you, including a more positive mindset, more energy, less inflammation and pain, and the ability to enjoy your surroundings along with the most important benefit, fighting stronger and living longer.

• APPENDIX •

Meal Plans

When going through the program, the toughest part is, *"What the heck can I make for dinner? What meals can I create using the principles listed in this book?"* This section has a combination of recipes to help you stick to the process in an easily divided format based on what step you are in the guide.

Below is a list of meal plans that you can individualize for your needs. Each meal plan includes proper nutrition as well as providing you the energy and fuel needed to fight breast cancer.

- **Seven Day Sample Meal Plan**
- **Seven day detox:** This diet includes recipes for following the seven day detox which is mentioned in chapter 9. This includes detox drinks, bone broth and soup recipes.
- **Hormone Balancing Diet:** This diet contains key ingredients to promote healthy sex hormone balance and detoxification, adrenal health, and thyroid function. Recipes include

the adaptogens maca and schisandra, as well as foods that support liver and gut health. Focus is on indole-3-carbinol, calcium-d-glucarate, omega-3s, iodine, probiotics, and fibre, as well as regular meals and plenty of protein for balanced blood sugar.

- **A Plant-Based Meal Plan:** This plan offers balanced nutrition without the use of animal products. The Whole Food Plant Based Diet is a completely animal product-free approach to healthy eating that maximizes whole grains, vegetables and legumes, while minimizing refined sugars and oils. This plan provides adequate protein from a variety of plant-based sources including grains, legumes, nuts and seeds. Fats are provided by whole food sources like avocados, nuts/seeds, and high-quality oils.

- **Ketogenic Meal Plan for Breast Cancer:** A high fat diet, low-carb meal plan to kick the body from glucose dependency into ketosis. Included is a wide range of nutrient-dense, high-fibre ingredients. The majority of carbohydrates on this plan come from fibre, so they will not prevent ketosis. They will, however, support a healthy gastrointestinal tract and make for a stronger and healthier immune system.

SEVEN DAY SAMPLE MEAL PLAN

(incorporated intermittent fasting 16/8 guidelines)

*All recipes for the 7 day sample meal plan are included in the Recipe Index.

Day 1

8:00am: Warm Water - 500mL

10:00am: Lucky Green Smoothie & 1/2 cup Mixed Almonds, Walnuts, Brazil nuts

1:00pm: Mexican Black Bean Salad

6:00pm: Halibut and Dill Pesto and Bone Broth Soup

Day 2

8:00am: Warm Water - 500mL

10:00am: Kale and Eggs Plus Green Juice

1:00pm: Butternut Squash Soup topped with 1 Tbsp each of Hemp, Flax, Sesame Seeds

6:00pm: Baked Salmon with Broccoli and Quinoa

Day 3

8:00am: Warm Water - 500mL

10:00am: Eggvocado Plus Blueberry Protein
Smoothie

1:00pm: Broccoli Soup Plus 1Tbsp each of
Ground Flax, and Chia Seeds

6:00pm: Slow Cooker Cabbage Roll Soup

Day 4

8:00am: Warm Water - 500mL

10:00am: Chocolate Cauliflower Shake

1:00pm: Protein Packed Deviled Eggs Plus
Bone Broth

6:00pm: Slow Cooker Cod and Sea Veggie
Soup

Day 5

8:00am: Warm Water - 500mL

10:00am: Overnight Vanilla Protein Oats

1:00pm: Avocado Toast with Poached Egg Plus
Bone Broth Soup

6:00pm: Balsamic Roasted Tempeh Bowl

Day 6

8:00am: Warm Water - 500mL

10:00am: Berry Beet Smoothie Bowl

1:00pm: Roasted Sweet Potato & Brussel Sprouts Salad

6:00pm: Slow Cooker Lentil Chili

Day 7

8:00am: Warm Water - 500mL

10:00am: Grain Free Coconut Almond Porridge

1:00pm: Creamy Cauliflower and Carrot Soup

6:00pm: Swiss Chard, Lentil and Rice Bowl

RECIPE INDEX:[1]

*All recipes were created, modified and extracted with the assistance of Thatcleanlife.com

SEVEN DAY DETOX RECIPES
SECTION 1: DRINKS and BONE BROTH

1.1-Detox Drink 1:
Ingredients:
- 1 tbsp. Clean Bowels
- 250mL of Filtered Water
- 1 Tbsp Olive Oil
- 20 Drops of Bio Cell Salts
- 1 Scoop of amino acid powder

1.2-Detox Drink 2:
Ingredients:
- 1 tbsp. of Organic Apple Cider Vinegar
- 1 cup Filtered Water

1.3-Green Juice:
Ingredients:
- 4 Stalks of Celery
- 6 Dandelion Leaves
- 1 Large Cucumber
- ½ Peeled Lemon
- 1 inch Peeled Ginger
- 2 Granny Smith Apples

1. Press organic ingredients through juicer, and drink within 24 hours - 2 servings

1.4-Pressure Cooker Bone Broth
Ingredients:
- 1 Whole Chicken Carcass
- 2 Carrots (medium, chopped)
- 1 Yellow Onion (chopped)

1 tbsp. Apple Cider Vinegar
1 tsp. Sea Salt
5 cups Water

1. Add the cooked chicken carcass/bones to the pressure cooker along with the carrots, onion, apple cider vinegar and sea salt.
2. Add the water to the pressure cooker. Lock the lid on and make sure the knob is set to the "sealing" position. Select the "manual" or "pressure cook" (on newer models) setting and set for two hours.
3. Once the two hours are up, allow the pressure to release naturally. Then open the lid carefully and strain the broth through a sieve or strainer. Discard the veggies and bones then transfer the broth into jars. Enjoy!

SECTION 2: SOUPS

2.1-Broccoli Soup

Ingredients:
1 tsp Avocado Oil
½ Yellow Onion (chopped)
2-3 Garlic (cloves, minced)
2 tbsp Arrowroot Powder
3 cups Organic Chicken Broth
1 cup Organic Coconut Milk (full fat, from a can)
4 cups Broccoli (florets, roughly chopped)
¼ cup Nutritional Yeast
¼ tsp Sea Salt

1. In a large pot over medium heat, add the avocado oil and then the onion. Cook for 3 to 4 minutes or until the onion becomes translucent. Add the garlic and cook for one minute. Add the arrowroot powder and chicken broth and whisk until no clumps remain.
2. Bring to a boil over medium heat, and then reduce to a simmer. Add the coconut milk, broccoli, nutritional yeast and salt and stir to combine. Cook for 10 minutes or until the broccoli is cooked through.
3. Using a handheld blender, blend the soup until smooth or until desired consistency is reached. Serve and enjoy!

2.2-Butternut Squash Soup

Ingredients:
    ½ Butternut Squash
    ½ tsp. Cinnamon
    1 tbsp. Extra Virgin Olive Oil (divided)
    ½ tbsp. Ginger (grated)
    2 cups Organic Vegetable Broth
    1 tsp. Sea Salt (divided)
    1/16 tsp. Cayenne Pepper

1. Put squash into a steamer for approximately 20 minutes, until soft.
2. Cut open and use a spoon to carve out the flesh and set aside. Discard the skin.
3. Place a large pot over medium heat, add in vegetable broth, cooked squash, sea salt and cayenne pepper. Reduce heat to a simmer.
4. Transfer soup to a blender or use an immersion

blender to puree until the soup reaches a smooth, thick consistency.

2.3-Pressure Cooker Carrot Ginger Soup

Ingredients:

3 cups Organic Vegetable Broth
1 Yellow Onion (chopped)
1 Garlic (clove, minced)
1 tbsp Ginger (fresh, minced)
6 Carrots (chopped)
2 tsp Thyme (fresh, chopped)
1¼ cups Organic Coconut Milk (full fat, from a can)

1. Sauté a splash of vegetable broth along with the onion and cook for 3 to 4 minutes. Add the garlic and ginger and sauté for 1 minute more.
2. Turn the sauté mode off and add the carrots, thyme and rest of the broth. Put the lid on and set to "sealing" then press the manual/pressure cooker and cook for 5 minutes on high pressure. Once finished, release the pressure manually.
3. Carefully remove the lid, and purée the soup using an immersion blender or a blender. Add the coconut milk and stir to combine. Serve and enjoy!

2.4-Celery Soup

Serving Size

One serving is approximately 2 cups.

Ingredients:

3 cups Organic Vegetable Broth (divided)

1 White Onion (diced)

1 Purple Potato (medium, diced)

12 stalks of Celery (diced, leaves reserved)

½ tsp Sea Salt

*More Flavor

Add dill and/or coconut milk to the soup.

1. In a large pot over medium heat, add a small splash of the vegetable broth. Sauté the onions until soft and brown, stirring frequently and adding more broth as needed to prevent the onions from sticking to the pot.

2. Add the potato, diced celery stalk, remaining broth and sea salt. Bring to a simmer and cook for 10 minutes or until the potatoes and celery are tender.

3. Use a handheld blender to purée to your desired consistency. Divide into bowls or containers. Top with celery leaves and enjoy!

2.5-Pumpkin Soup

Ingredients:

2 tbsp Coconut Oil

2 ¼ cups Pureed Pumpkin

2 cups Organic Vegetable Broth

½ cup Unsweetened Almond Milk

1 tsp Ground Ginger

1 tsp Ground Sage

1 ½ tsp Maple Syrup

½ tsp Sea Salt

¼ tsp Black Pepper

¼ cup Organic Coconut Milk (optional)

1. In a large pot, heat coconut oil over medium heat. Stir in pumpkin, broth, almond milk, ginger, sage, maple syrup, salt and pepper.
2. Bring to a boil and let simmer for about 10 minutes

HORMONE BALANCING DIET RECIPES
SECTION 1: SHAKES AND SMOOTHIES AND DRINKS

1.1- Chocolate Cauliflower Shake
Ingredients:
- 2 cups Frozen Cauliflower
- 2 Banana (frozen)
- 2 tbsp. Almond Butter
- ¼ cup Cacao Powder
- ½ cup Chocolate Protein Powder
- 2 cups Unsweetened Almond Milk
- 1 tbsp. Maca Powder

1. In your blender, combine all ingredients. Blend until smooth, pour into glasses and enjoy!

1.2-Berry Beet Smoothie Bowl
Ingredients:
- 1 ½ Beets (medium, peeled and diced)
- 1 ½ cups Frozen Mango
- 1 ½ cups Frozen Raspberries
- 1 ½ tbsp. Pitted Dates
- 1 ½ tsp. Schisandra Berry Powder
- 1 ½ cups Unsweetened Almond Milk

1. In your blender or food processor, combine the beets, frozen mango, frozen raspberries, dates, schisandra berry powder and milk. Blend until smooth and thick.
2. Transfer to a bowl and add toppings. Enjoy!

1.3-Bloat Fighting Tropical Smoothie

Ingredients:

½ cup Papaya (chopped)
½ cup Pineapple (chopped)
½ Cucumber (chopped)
2 ½ Ice Cubes
¼ cup Mint Leaves
½ cup Baby Spinach
1 tbsp Chia Seeds
½ cup Water

1.   Add all ingredients to the blender and blend until smooth.
2.   Pour into a glass and enjoy!

1.4-Blueberry Protein Smoothie

Ingredients:

¼ cup Vanilla Protein Powder
1 tbsp. Ground Flax Seed
1 cup Frozen Blueberries
1 cup Baby Spinach
1 cup Water (cold)

1. Throw all ingredients into a blender and blend until smooth. Pour into a glass and enjoy!

1.5-Detox Green Smoothie

Ingredients:

4 cups Kale Leaves
1 Cucumber (chopped)
1 Lemon (juiced)
2 Pears (peeled and chopped)
1 tbsp. Ginger (grated)

1 tbsp. Ground Flax Seeds
1 ½ cup Water
5 Ice Cubes

1. Throw all ingredients together in a blender. Blend until smooth. Be patient! No one likes clumps in their smoothies. It may take 1 minute or longer to get a great, smoothie-consistency.
2. Divide between glasses and enjoy!

1.6-Lucky Green Smoothie
Ingredients:
    1 ½ cups Frozen Mango
    2 Lime (juiced)
    2 cups Baby Spinach (packed)
    2 tbsp. Ground Flax Seeds
    ¼ cup Hemp Seeds
    3 ½ cups Water

1. Throw all ingredients into a blender. Blend well until smooth. Divide into glasses and enjoy!

1.7-Pressure Cooker Bone Broth
Ingredients:
    1 Whole Chicken Carcass
    2 Carrots (medium, chopped)
    1 Yellow Onion (chopped)
    1 tbsp. Apple Cider Vinegar
    1 tsp. Sea Salt
    5 cups Water

1. Add the cooked chicken carcass/bones to the pressure cooker along with the carrots, onion,

apple cider vinegar and sea salt.

2. Add the water to the pressure cooker. Lock the lid on and make sure the knob is set to the "sealing" position. Select the "manual" or "pressure cook" (on newer models) setting and set for two hours.

3. Once the two hours are up, allow the pressure to release naturally. Then open the lid carefully and strain the broth through a sieve or strainer. Discard the veggies and bones then transfer the broth into jars. Enjoy!

SECTION 2: SNACKS AND MEALS

2.1–Grain Free Coconut Almond Porridge

Ingredients:
¾ cup Unsweetened Almond Milk
¼ cup Almond Flour
¼ cup Unsweetened Shredded Coconut
1 tbsp. Ground Flax Seeds
½ tsp. Cinnamon

1. Add all of the ingredients to a saucepan over medium heat. Whisk continuously until your desired thickness is reached, about 3 to 5 minutes.

2. Divide into bowls and enjoy!

2.2–Overnight Vanilla Protein Oats

Ingredients:
1 cup Oats (quick or traditional)
1 tbsp. Chia Seeds
1 ¼ cup Unsweetened Almond Milk

270

¼ cup Vanilla Protein Powder

¼ cup Raspberries

¼ cup Blueberries

1 tbsp. Almond Butter

1. In a large bowl or container combine the oats, chia seeds and milk. Stir to combine. Place in the fridge for 8 hours, or overnight.
2. After the oats have set, remove from the fridge and add the protein powder. Mix well. Add extra almond milk 1 tbsp at a time if the oats are too thick.
3. Divide the oats into bowls or containers and top with raspberries, blueberries and almond butter. Enjoy!

2.3–Plaintain Coconut Fritters

Ingredients:

2 Plantains (unripe, peeled and sliced)

¼ cup Coconut Oil (melted)

½ tsp. Sea Salt

½ cup Unsweetened Coconut Yogurt

1 tbsp. Dried Chives

1. Preheat the oven to 375F (190C). Line a baking sheet with parchment paper or a silicone baking mat.
2. Add the plantain, coconut oil and sea salt to a food processor or blender. Blend into a thick puree.
3. Use a spoon to scoop the batter onto the baking sheet and spread out to approximately two inches wide and half-inch thick.

4. Bake until the fritters begin to brown around edges, about 15 to 20 minutes. Serve with coconut yogurt and chives. Enjoy!

2.4-Slow Cooker Cod and Sea Veggie Soup
Ingredients:
   3 tbsp. Coconut Oil
   1 Yellow Onion (medium, diced)
   4 cup Mushrooms (sliced)
   3 Garlic (cloves, minced)
   3 tbsp. Ginger (peeled and grated)
   1 1/3 ounces Dulse (torn apart into small pieces)
   2 Sweet Potatoes (medium, diced)
   4 Cod Fillets (cubed)
   8 cup Organic Vegetable Broth (or bone broth)

1. Heat the coconut oil in a frying pan over medium heat. Add the onion and mushrooms. Saute for about 3 minutes or until onions are translucent. Add garlic and ginger. Cook for 1 to 2 minutes until fragrant.
2. Transfer the contents of the pan to your slow cooker. Add the dulse (ripped into bite-sized pieces), diced sweet potato, cod and broth. Do not add salt, as the dulse is naturally very salty and should flavour the soup.
3. Cook on high for 4 hours, or low for 6 to 8 hours. Taste, and add sea salt if necessary.
4. Divide between bowls and enjoy!

2.5- Creamy Cauliflower and Carrot Soup
Ingredients:
   2 tbsp. Extra Virgin Olive Oil

6 stalks Green Onion (chopped)
5 Carrots (medium size, chopped)
1 head Cauliflower (chopped into florets)
6 cups Water
2 tsp. Dried Thyme
½ tsp. Sea Salt
½ cup Parsley

1. Heat the olive oil in a large stock pot over medium-low heat. Add the green onions and saute until softened. Add the carrots, cauliflower, water, thyme and salt. Cover the pot and bring to a boil. Once boiling, reduce to a simmer. Let simmer for 20 minutes then add in the parsley and stir until wilted. Turn off the heat.

2. Puree the soup using a blender or handheld immersion blender. (Note: If using a regular blender, be careful. Ensure you leave a space for the steam to escape.) Taste and adjust seasoning if needed. Ladle into bowls and enjoy!

2.6- Slow Cooker Cabbage Roll Soup
Ingredients:
1 head Cauliflower (processed into rice)
4 cups Green Cabbage (roughly chopped)
1 Yellow Onion (diced)
4 Garlic (cloves, minced)
3 cups Crushed Tomatoes
1 tbsp. Extra Virgin Olive Oil
2 tbsp. Italian Seasoning
½ tsp. Red Pepper Flakes (optional)
1 tsp. Sea Salt & Black Pepper

1 cup Water

1 pound Extra Lean Ground Turkey (or chicken)

4 cups Baby Spinach

1/3 cup Parsley (chopped, optional)

1. Use a food processor to pulse your cauliflower into rice.
2. Add all ingredients except ground turkey, spinach and parsley to your slow cooker. Stir very well to combine. Set ground turkey on the top. Cover with a lid. Cook on low for 7 to 8 hours or on high for 4 hours (or until meat is fully cooked through).
3. Before serving, take the lid off and use a wooden spoon to break the cooked ground turkey into small pieces. Stir in the spinach until wilted. Ladle into bowls and garnish with parsley. Enjoy!

2.7- Mexican Black Bean Salad

Ingredients:

2 cups Black Beans (cooked)

1 Red Bell Pepper (chopped)

¼ cup Red Onion (chopped)

1 Avocado (diced)

¼ cup Lime Juice

¼ tsp. Chili Powder

¼ tsp.Cumin

1/8 tsp.Sea Salt

1. In a large mixing bowl combine the black beans, pepper, onion and avocado.
2. Add the lime juice, chili powder, cumin, and

salt to a mason jar. Seal with a lid and shake until combined. Pour dressing over the black bean mixture and stir until evenly coated.

3. Serve chilled and enjoy.

2.8- Parchment Baked Haddock with Veggies

Ingredients:

2 cups Green Beans (trimmed)

1 Red Bell Pepper (thinly sliced)

3 stalks Green Onion (green parts only, chopped)

2 Haddock Fillets (5 ounces each)

1 tbsp. Extra Virgin Olive Oil

1 Lemon (zested and juiced)

¼ tsp. Sea Salt

¼ tsp. Black Pepper

1 tbsp. Fresh Dill

1. Preheat your oven to 400F (204C). Cut pieces of parchment paper, about 18-inches long. You'll need one per fillet of fish. Fold each piece of parchment in half then unfold.

2. Divide the green beans, peppers and green onion equally between parchment pieces, placing the vegetables neatly on the right side of the parchment paper. Place one haddock fillet on top of each portion of vegetables.

3. Drizzle the olive oil, lemon juice and lemon zest over top of each fillet. Season each portion equally with salt, pepper and dill.

4. Fold the other side of the parchment paper over the fish and the veggies. Starting at one side, crimp and fold the edges of the parchment together to tightly seal the packets. Carefully

transfer the parchment packets to a baking sheet.

5. Bake for 16 to 19 minutes, or until haddock flakes easily and is cooked through. (To check doneness, very carefully unfold one side of the parchment packet and check to see if the fish flakes with a fork. If it isn't done yet, fold it back up and continue baking.)

6. To serve, transfer the parchment to a plate and very carefully cut into the top of the packet. Enjoy!

2.9- Protein Packed Deviled Eggs

Ingredients:

4 Eggs (hard boiled)

1 can of flaked Tuna (drained)

½ Avocado

1 stalk Green Onion (chopped)

Sea Salt & Black Pepper (to taste)

½ tsp. Paprika

½ Cucumber (sliced)

1. Hard boil your eggs.

2. Once cool, peel the eggs and slice them in half. Remove the yolk and add it to a bowl.

3. Add in the tuna, avocado and green onion. Season with sea salt and black pepper to taste. Mix and mash very well and then stuff the mixture back into the eggs.

4. Sprinkle it with paprika and enjoy with cucumber slices on the side.

2.10- Avocado Toast with a Poached Egg

Ingredients:

1 slice Organic Bread
½ Avocado
Sea Salt & Black Pepper (to taste)
1 Egg
1 tbsp. Apple Cider Vinegar
1/8 tsp. Sea Salt

1. Toast bread.
2. Cut avocado in half, remove the pit and cut into fine slices. Layer avocado on the toast, mash with a fork and season with a bit of sea salt and black pepper.
3. Crack your egg into a bowl.
4. Bring a pot of water to a rolling boil on your stovetop. Add sea salt and vinegar. Begin stirring your water with a spoon to create a whirlpool. Carefully add your egg into the whirlpool. Cook for 3 to 4 minutes then use a slotted spoon to carefully remove from the hot water. Place the poached egg onto a plate lined with a paper towel to soak up the excess liquid.
5. Transfer the egg to the top of your toast and season again with sea salt and pepper. Enjoy!

2.11- Roasted Sweet Potato & Brussel Sprouts Salad

Ingredients:

1 ½ Sweet Potato (medium sliced into 1 inch cubes)
3 cups Brussels Sprouts (washed and halved)
2 ¼ tsp. Extra Virgin Olive Oil

Sea Salt & Black Pepper (to taste)

3 tbsp. Tahini

2 ¼ tsps. Maple Syrup

3 tbsp. Water (warm)

1/8 tsp. Cayenne Pepper (less if you don't like it spicy)

1/16 tsp. Sea Salt

1 ½ cups Lentils (cooked, drained and rinsed)

6 cups Spinach (chopped)

1. Preheat the oven to 425F (218C). Line a large baking sheet with parchment paper.

2. Combine the diced sweet potato and brussels sprouts in a bowl. Add olive oil and season with sea salt and black pepper to taste. Toss well then spread across the baking sheet. Bake in the oven for 30 minutes or until both vegetables are cooked through and starting to brown.

3. While the vegetables roast, combine the tahini, maple syrup, water, cayenne pepper and sea salt in a jar. Seal with a lid and shake well to mix. Set aside.

4. Remove the roasted vegetables from the oven and place back in the mixing bowl. Add in the lentils. Mix well.

5. Divide spinach between bowls. Top with lentils and roasted vegetable mix. Drizzle with the desired amount of dressing. Enjoy!

2.12- Almonds and Dark Chocolate

Ingredients:

3 ½ ounces Dark Organic Chocolate (at least 70% cacao)

½ cup Almonds

1. Divide between bowls. Enjoy!

2.13- Egg Roll in a Bowl

Ingredients:

1 tbsp. Avocado Oil

½ Yellow Onion (medium, diced)

2 ½ stalks Green Onion (diced)

2 Garlic (cloves, minced)

1 ½ tsp. Ginger (peeled and grated)

8 ounces Lean Ground Pork

3 cups Coleslaw Mix

1 cup Bean Sprouts

2 tbsp Coconut Aminos

1. Heat the avocado oil in a pan over medium-high heat. Add the yellow onion, green onion, garlic, and ginger. Cook for 3 to 5 minutes, stirring frequently, until soft.
2. Add the pork and break it up as it cooks. Cook for about 7 to 10 minutes, or until cooked through.
3. Stir in the coleslaw mix, bean sprouts, and coconut aminos. Stir for 5 minutes, or until veggies have softened. Transfer to bowls and enjoy!

2.14– Halibut and Dill Pesto

Ingredients:

½ cup Parsley (packed)

2 tbsp. Fresh Dill (packed)

2 2/3 tbsp. Slivered Almonds

1 ½ tbsp. Extra Virgin Olive Oil

½ Lemon (juiced)

½ Garlic (clove)

Sea Salt & Black Pepper (to taste)

10 ounce Halibut Fillet

¾ tsp. Coconut Oil

4 cups Mixed Greens (or Arugula)

1. In a food processor, combine the parsley, dill, slivered almonds, olive oil, lemon juice and garlic. Season with sea salt and black pepper to taste and blend well until a thick paste forms. Transfer to a bowl and set aside.

2. Season halibut with sea salt and black pepper. Heat coconut oil in a cast iron skillet over medium-high heat. Cook fish for 3 to 4 minutes per side, or until golden. Fish should flake with a fork when finished.

3. Divide mixed greens between plates. Set halibut on the greens and top with a large dollop of pesto. Enjoy!

2.15– Sausage and Sauerkraut Skillet

Ingredients:

5 ounces Organic Chicken Sausage

1 ½ tsp. Coconut Oil

½ Yellow Onion (diced)

1 Apple (peeled, cored and diced)

1 Garlic (clove, minced)

2 cups Swiss Chard (washed, stems removed and chopped)

1 cup Sauerkraut (liquid drained off)

1. Preheat the oven to 350F (177C). Line a baking sheet with parchment paper. Add sausage and bake for 30 minutes or until cooked through. Remove from the oven and cut into 1/4" pieces.

2. Heat coconut oil in a frying pan over medium heat. Add yellow onion and apple. Saute just until the onion is translucent (about 5 minutes). Add garlic and saute for another minute.

3. Add swiss chard and continue to saute just until it is wilted. Reduce heat to low and add in chopped sausage and sauerkraut and saute for another minute or until heated through. Remove from heat and divide into bowls.

2.16–Slow Cooker Lentil Chili

Ingredients:

1 cup Dry Red Lentils (rinsed, uncooked)

1 Yellow Onion (medium, diced)

1 Red Bell Pepper (chopped)

1 Carrot (chopped)

3 Garlic (cloves, minced)

1 tbsp. Chili Powder

1 tsp. Cumin

1 tsp. Smoked Paprika

3 ½ cups Diced Tomatoes (from the can with juices)

2 tbsp. Tomato Paste

2 cups Organic Vegetable Broth

Sea Salt & Black Pepper (to taste)

1 ¾ cups Red Kidney Beans (from the can, drained and rinsed)

1 Avocado (optional, sliced)

¼ cup Cilantro (optional, chopped)

1. Add lentils, onion, bell pepper, carrot, garlic, chili powder, cumin, paprika, tomatoes, tomato paste, vegetable broth, sea salt and pepper to your slow cooker. Stir well to combine.

2. Cover and cook on low for 6 to 7 hours, depending on the strength of your slow cooker. Once it is cooked through, add the kidney beans and stir to combine.

3. Ladle into bowls and top with avocado and cilantro (optional). Enjoy!

2.17- Baked Salmon with Broccoli and Quinoa

Ingredients:

15 ounces Salmon Fillets

Sea Salt & Black Pepper (to taste)

6 cups Broccoli (sliced into small florets)

1 ½ tbsp. Extra Virgin Olive Oil

¾ cup Quinoa (uncooked)

1 1/8 cup Water

1/3 Lemon (sliced into wedges)

1. Preheat the oven to 450F (232C) and line a baking sheet with parchment paper.

2. Place the salmon fillets on the baking sheet and season with sea salt and black pepper.

3. Toss the broccoli florets in olive oil and season with sea salt and black pepper. Add them to

the baking sheet, arranging them around the salmon fillets. Bake the salmon and broccoli in the oven for 15 minutes, or until the salmon flakes with a fork.

4. While the salmon cooks, combine the quinoa and water together in a saucepan. Bring to a boil over high heat, then reduce to a simmer. Cover and let simmer for 12 to 15 minutes, or until all water is absorbed. Remove the lid and fluff with a fork. Set aside.

5. Remove the salmon and broccoli from the oven and divide onto plates. Serve with quinoa and a lemon wedge. Season with extra sea salt, black pepper and olive oil if you like. Enjoy!

2.18- Fish Tacos with Pineapple Salsa

Ingredients:

4 Brown Rice Tortillas (thawed)
2 Tilapia Fillets
1 1/2 tsp. Extra Virgin Olive Oil
Sea Salt & Black Pepper (to taste)
1 Lemon (juiced)
1 cup Baby Spinach
½ cup Pineapple (diced)
½ cup Red Onion (finely diced)
1 Jalapeno Pepper (deseeded and chopped)
1 Garlic (clove, minced)
1 Red Bell Pepper (diced)
1 Lime (juiced)
2 Avocado (peeled and mashed)
1 Tomato (diced)

1. Preheat the oven to 500F (260C) and move the rack to the top setting. Cover a large baking sheet with parchment paper and lightly grease with some olive oil. Lightly rub white fish with extra virgin olive oil, a splash of lemon juice and season with sea salt and pepper. Cook in the oven on top rack for 8 minutes or until fish flakes with a fork.

2. Remove fish from the oven and chop with a knife. Place in a bowl and toss with a bit of lemon juice.

3. Prepare all ingredients for the salsa and mix together in a large mixing bowl. (Pineapple, red onion, jalapeno, red bell pepper, and lime juice).

4. Prepare all ingredients for the guacamole and mix together in a separate mixing bowl. (Avocado, tomato, garlic and splash of lemon juice).

5. Warm your tortillas and place on a plate. Put your salsa, guacamole, spinach and fish out in separate bowls with a spoon/fork in each. Happy fish taco night!

2.19– Swiss Chard, Lentil and Rice Bowl

Ingredients:

½ cup Brown Rice (uncooked)

¾ cup Water

1 tbsp. Coconut Oil

8 cups Swiss Chard (washed, stems removed and chopped)

1 tsp. Cumin

1 tsp. Paprika

2 tbsp. Extra Virgin Olive Oil
1 Garlic (clove, minced)
1 tbsp. Apple Cider Vinegar
2 cups Lentils (cooked, drained and rinsed)
Sea Salt & Black Pepper (to taste)

1. Combine the rice and water in a medium sized pot and lightly salt the water. Bring to a boil over medium-high heat then reduce to a simmer. Cover the pot and let cook for 40 to 50 minutes or until rice is tender.
2. Heat a large skillet over medium heat and add the coconut oil. Add the swiss chard and saute just until wilted. Reduce the heat to low and stir in the cumin, paprika, olive oil, garlic, apple cider vinegar and lentils. Stir well until everything is well mixed. Add in the rice once it is cooked, and continue to saute. Season with sea salt and black pepper to taste. Divide into bowls and enjoy!

2.20–Vegan Sloppy Joe
Ingredients:
4 cups Lentils (cooked, drained and rinsed)
½ Sweet Onion (finely diced)
1 Green Bell Pepper (finely diced)
2 cups Mushrooms (sliced)
1 cup Matchstick Carrots
1 tbsp. Garlic Powder
3 tbsp. Yellow Mustard
¼ cup Maple Syrup
2 cups Crushed Tomatoes
1 tsp. Sea Salt

½ tsp. Black Pepper
1 ½ lbs.Portobello Mushroom Caps
2 cup Baby Spinach (chopped)

1. Combine the lentils, onion, green pepper, mushrooms, carrots, garlic powder, yellow mustard, maple syrup, crushed tomatoes, sea salt and black pepper in the slow cooker. Use a spatula to mix well. Cover and cook on high for 4 hours or on low for 6 hours.

2. About 20 minutes before you are ready to eat, preheat your oven to 400 and line a baking sheet with parchment paper. Place your portobello mushroom caps on a baking sheet and bake for 10 minutes.

3. Place a portobello mushroom cap on a plate and top with a few large spoonfuls of the sloppy joe mix. Top with baby spinach and set another mushroom cap on top. Enjoy!

WHOLE FOODS PLANT BASED MEAL PLAN RECIPES
SECTION 1- SMOOTHIES

1.1- Gut Healing Green Smoothie
Ingredients:
- 1 ¼ cup Water (cold)
- 1 cup Kale Leaves
- ¼ Avocado (peeled and pit removed)
- ½ Banana (frozen)
- 1 ½ tsp. Chia Seeds
- 1 tbsp. Ground Flax Seed
- 2 tbsp. Hemp Seeds
- 1 tbsp. Raw Honey

1. Throw all ingredients into a blender and blend until very smooth and creamy. Divide into glasses and enjoy!

SECTION 2-SNACKS and MEALS

SNACKS include any of the following delicious options:
- ☆ 1 cup of pistachios
- ☆ 2 cups of grapes with ½ cup of walnuts
- ☆ ¼ cup of Brazilian nuts
- ☆ 1 apple with a ¼ cup of hummus
- ☆ 2 ¼ cups of baby carrots with ¼ cup of hummus

2.1- Protein Packed Avocado Toast

Ingredients:

½ Avocado
½ cup White Navy Beans (cooked)
1/8 Lemon (juiced)
1/8 tsp. Sea Salt
2 slices of Organic Bread
2 tbsp. Hemp Seeds

1. In a bowl, mash the avocado, white beans, lemon juice and sea salt together with a fork. Continue to mash until you get a guacamole-like consistency.
2. Divide the avocado bean mixture onto the toast. Sprinkle with hemp seeds and enjoy!

2.2- Hummus Toast with Avocado

Ingredients:

2 slices Rye Bread (toasted)
½ cup Hummus
½ Avocado (sliced or mashed)
2 tbsp. Sunflower Seeds
Sea Salt & Black Pepper (to taste)

1. Spread hummus over toast and top with avocado slices, sunflower seeds, salt and pepper. Enjoy!

2.3- Tofu Veggie Scramble

Ingredients:

7 ¾ cups Tofu (firm)
1 tbsp. Avocado Oil
½ Yellow Onion (medium, diced)
2 Garlic (cloves, minced)

1 Red Bell Pepper (sliced)
1 cup Baby Spinach (chopped)
1 tbsp. Nutritional Yeast
¼ tsp. Turmeric
Sea Salt & Black Pepper (to taste)

1. Place the tofu in a small bowl and mash with a fork to the point where it is broken apart but chunks still remain. The texture should be similar to scrambled eggs.
2. In a non-stick pan, heat the avocado oil over medium heat. Add the onions, garlic and bell pepper. Saute for 4 to 5 minutes, or until onions are translucent.
3. Add the tofu, spinach, nutritional yeast and turmeric to the pan. Mix well and cook until the spinach wilts and the tofu is heated through.
4. Season with sea salt and black pepper taste. Enjoy!

2.4– Marinated Mix Bean Salad

Ingredients:
1 ½ cups Green Beans (fresh or frozen)
3 cups Mixed Beans (cooked)
3 tbsp. Extra Virgin Olive Oil
1 ½ tbsp. Apple Cider Vinegar
2 ¼ tsp. Italian Seasoning
¾ Garlic (clove, minced)
¾ Lemon (juiced)
Sea Salt & Black Pepper (to taste)

1. Bring a medium-sized pot of salted water to a boil. Drop in the green beans and simmer for 3

to 5 minutes. Drain and rinse with cold water until cool.

2. Combine all ingredients together in a large mixing bowl. Toss well and enjoy right away, or let marinate in the fridge overnight for more flavour.

2.5– Broccoli Almond Protein Salad

Ingredients:

2 cups Broccoli (chopped into small florets)
1 cup Frozen Edamame (shelled)
2 stalks Green Onion (sliced)
¼ cup Almonds (chopped)
2 tbsp. Almond Butter
1 ½ tsp. Rice Vinegar
1 ½ tsp. Tamari (or Coconut Aminos)
1 ½ tsp. Maple Syrup
1 ½ tsp. Sesame Oil
½ Garlic (clove, minced)
1 tbsp. Water

1. In a large mixing bowl, combine the broccoli florets, edamame beans, green onions, and chopped almonds.

2. To make the salad dressing, whisk together the almond butter, rice vinegar, tamari, maple syrup, sesame oil, garlic, and water. Add more water if needed to achieve desired consistency.

3. Pour the dressing over the salad and toss to mix well. Serve immediately, or let sit for a few hours before eating. Enjoy!

2.6- Peanut Butter Curry Chickpea Stew

Ingredients:

1 ½ tsp. Coconut Oil
½ Yellow Onion (medium, diced)
1 Garlic (cloves, minced)
1 ½ tsp. Ginger (grated)
½ tsp. Cumin
½ tsp. Coriander
½ tsp. Cinnamon
1 ½ tsp. Turmeric
2 tbsp. Water
2 tbsp. All Natural Peanut Butter
1 cup Organic Vegetable Broth
½ cup Unsweetened Almond Milk
½ tsp. Sea Salt
½ Red Bell Pepper (sliced)
½ Zucchini (sliced)
1 Carrot (medium, peeled and sliced)
2 cups Chickpeas (cooked)
½ Lime (juiced)
2 tbsp. Cilantro (chopped)

1. Heat a large saucepan over medium-low heat and melt the coconut oil. Add the onion, garlic and ginger. Cook for 2-3 minutes, stirring frequently.
2. Add the spices and cook for 1 minute, until fragrant. Add the water to deglaze the pan, then stir in the peanut butter.
3. Add the vegetable broth and almond milk. Stir until all is smoothly combined. Add the salt.
4. Add the pepper, zucchini, carrots and chickpeas and stir well to mix. Simmer uncovered for 20

minutes, stirring occasionally.

5. Stir in the lime juice and cilantro. Divide into bowls, and top with more cilantro if desired. Enjoy!

2.7- Sweet Potato Black Bean Quinoa Bake

Ingredients:

1/3 cup Quinoa (dry, uncooked)
1 Sweet Potato (peeled, small pieces)
2/3 cups Black Beans (rinsed, from can)
1/3 Red Bell Pepper (chopped)
1 stalk Green Onion (chopped)
1 tsp. Chili Powder
1 tsp. Cumin (ground)
1/3 tsp. Garlic Powder
1/16 tsp. Sea Salt
2/3 cups Organic Vegetable Broth
1/3 Lime (juiced)
1/3 Avocado (diced)

1. Preheat the oven to 375°F (190°C).
2. In a large baking dish, add the sweet potatoes, black beans, quinoa, pepper, onion, chili powder, cumin, garlic and sea salt. Stir well to combine and then add the broth.
3. Cover the baking dish with foil and bake for 40 minutes or until the broth has absorbed completely, the quinoa is fluffy and the sweet potatoes are tender. Remove from the oven.
4. Let the quinoa bake sit for 5 minutes before dividing between plates. Top each plate with lime juice and avocado. Enjoy!

2.8-Lentil, Sweet Potato Salad

Ingredients:

1 Sweet Potato (medium, diced)
¾ tsp. Extra Virgin Olive Oil
2 tbsp. Tahini
2 tbsp. Water
1 ½ tsp. Maple Syrup
Sea Salt & Black Pepper (to taste)
2 cups Arugula
1 cup Lentils (cooked)

1. Preheat the oven to 425F (218C) and line a baking sheet with parchment paper.
2. Toss diced sweet potato in olive oil and spread across the baking sheet. Bake in the oven for 30 minutes, stirring at the halfway point.
3. Meanwhile, prepare the dressing by combining the tahini, water and maple syrup in a jar. Season with a pinch of sea salt and black pepper to taste. Seal with a lid and shake well to mix. Set aside.
4. Divide arugula into bowls and divide the lentils on top. Next, divide the roasted sweet potato between bowls. Drizzle with tahini dressing and enjoy!

2.9-Balsamic Roasted Tempeh Bowls

Ingredients:

1 1/3 tsps. Extra Virgin Olive Oil
1 1/3 tsps. Balsamic Vinegar
1 Garlic (clove, minced)
Sea Salt & Black Pepper (to taste)
1 tsp. Italian Seasoning

6 ounces Tempeh

1/3 cup Red Onion (medium, sliced)

2 Carrots (medium, peeled and chopped)

1 1/3 cup Mushrooms (quartered)

1 Zucchini (sliced)

½ cup Quinoa (dry)

¾ cup Water

1. Preheat the oven to 350F (177C).
2. Combine the olive oil, balsamic vinegar, garlic, sea salt, black pepper and Italian seasoning in a bowl and mix well. Place the tempeh, red onion, carrots, mushrooms and zucchini together in a large bowl and toss with the balsamic dressing to coat.
3. Transfer the veggies and tempeh to a large baking sheet and roast in the oven for 45 minutes, stirring halfway.
4. While the veggies and tempeh roast, make the quinoa. Bring the water to a boil in a small saucepan, add the quinoa, cover and simmer for 15 minutes. Remove from heat and fluff with a fork.
5. To serve, divide the quinoa between bowls and top with roasted veggies and tempeh. Garnish with additional balsamic vinegar if you'd like, and enjoy!

2.10-Swiss Chard & Lentil Rice Bowl

Ingredients:

2 tbsp. Brown Rice (uncooked)

3 tbsp. Water

¾ tbsp. Coconut Oil

2 cups Swiss Chard (washed, stems removed and chopped)
¼ tsp. Cumin
¼ tsp. Paprika
1 ½ tsp. Extra Virgin Olive Oil
¼ Garlic (clove, minced)
¾ tsp. Apple Cider Vinegar
½ cup Lentils (cooked, drained and rinsed)
Sea Salt & Black Pepper (to taste)

1. Combine the rice and water in a medium sized pot and lightly salt the water. Bring to a boil over medium-high heat then reduce to a simmer. Cover the pot and let cook for 40 to 50 minutes or until rice is tender.

2. Heat a large skillet over medium heat and add the coconut oil. Add the swiss chard and saute just until wilted. Reduce the heat to low and stir in the cumin, paprika, olive oil, garlic, apple cider vinegar and lentils. Stir well until everything is well mixed. Add in the rice once it is cooked, and continue to saute. Season with sea salt and black pepper to taste. Divide into bowls and enjoy!

KETOGENIC MEAL PLAN RECIPES
SECTION 1- DRINKS

1.1-Bulletproof Latte

Ingredients:

1 cup Organic Coffee (brewed)

1 tbsp. Ghee

2 tbsp. Organic Coconut Milk (canned, full-fat)

1. Pour your brewed coffee into a blender with the ghee and coconut milk. Blend on high for 15-30 seconds or until frothy. Pour into a mug and enjoy!

SECTION 2- SNACKS and MEALS

2.1-Eggvocado

Ingredients:

½ Avocado

1 Egg

1. Preheat the oven to 350F (177C).
2. Slice the avocado in half and scoop out a little flesh from each half to make room for the eggs. Place face-up on a baking sheet.
3. Crack an egg in each half of the avocado and bake for 10 to 15 minutes, depending on how runny you like your eggs. Enjoy!

2.2-Kale and Eggs

Ingredients:

½ tsp. Ghee

3 cups Kale Leaves (roughly chopped)

2 Eggs

2 tbsp. Pitted Kalamata Olives

1 tbsp. Nutritional Yeast

1/8 tsp. Sea Salt

1. Heat a skillet over medium heat and add the ghee. Once the skillet is hot, add the kale and cook for 2 to 3 minutes, until just wilted, stirring as needed.

2. Make two spaces in the kale and crack eggs into each space. Add the olives and season everything with nutritional yeast and sea salt. Cover with a lid and cook for 3 to 4 minutes or until the eggs are cooked to your preference.

3. Add the kale, olives and eggs to a plate. Serve and enjoy!

2.3-Smoked Salmon Wrapped Avocado

Ingredients:

1 Avocado

3 ½ ounces of Smoked Salmon

1. Slice the avocado and wrap each slice with the smoked salmon. Transfer to a plate and enjoy!

2.4-Olive Medley

Ingredients:

3 cups Assorted Olives

1. Divide into bowls and enjoy!

2.5–Tuna Salad Lettuce Wraps

Ingredients:

1 can Tuna (flaked)

1 Avocado

2 tbsp. Lime Juice

¼ tsp. Sea Salt

2 stalks Green Onion (sliced)

1/8 Cucumber (deseeded and finely chopped)

4 Leaves of Romaine

1. In a mixing bowl mash the avocado together with lime juice and salt. Stir in the tuna until well combined.
2. Fold in the green onion and cucumber. Season with additional salt and lime if needed. Divide the tuna salad between the romaine leaves and enjoy!

2.6–One Pan Mediterranean Trout

Ingredients:

1 cup Basil Leaves

¼ Lemon (juiced)

½ Garlic (clove)

1/8 tsp. Sea Salt

2 tbsp. Hemp Seeds

2 tbsp. Extra Virgin Olive Oil

2 Rainbow Trout Fillets (about 5 oz. each)

¾ cup Artichoke Hearts

¼ cup Pitted Kalamata Olives

1 Tomato (large, quartered)

1. Preheat the oven to 400F (204C) and line a baking sheet with parchment.

2. Make pesto by combining basil, lemon juice, garlic, sea salt, hemp seeds and olive oil together in a small food processor. Pulse until smooth.

3. Lay rainbow trout on a baking sheet and arrange the artichokes, olives and tomatoes on the baking dish around the fillets. Top each piece of trout with a generous spoonful of pesto.

4. Bake for 15 minutes or until fish is cooked through. Divide onto plates and enjoy!

2.7–Pesto Zoodles with Poached Egg

Ingredients:

2 Zucchini (large)
½ cup Basil Leaves
½ cup Baby Spinach
½ Garlic (clove, minced)
2 tbsp. Walnuts
2 ½ tbsp. Extra Virgin Olive Oil
½ Lemon (juiced)
¼ tsp. Sea Salt
2 Eggs

1. Spiralize your zucchini into "zoodles" and set aside.

2. In a food processor combine basil, spinach, garlic, walnuts, olive oil, lemon juice and sea salt. Blend until smooth.

3. Fry your eggs in a skillet or poach them in a small saucepan with water and vinegar. Transfer them to a plate lined with a paper towel.

4. You can serve this dish in two ways: For a cold dish, toss your zucchini noodles in the desired

amount of pesto, top with a fried or poached egg and serve. Or, for a warm dish, heat a bit of olive oil in the skillet and saute your noodles until warmed through, add pesto and work it around with tongs to evenly distribute. Transfer to bowls and top with a fried egg. Enjoy!

2.8–Sausage, Broccoli and Cabbage Stir Fry

Ingredients:
   5 ounces Organic Chicken Sausage
   ½ Yellow Onion (small, diced)
   ½ Garlic (clove, minced)
   2 cups Broccoli (chopped into small florets)
   2 cups Purple Cabbage (finely sliced)
   1 tsp. Italian Seasoning

1. Remove casings from the sausage and discard. Heat a large skillet over medium-high heat. Add the sausage meat, onion, and garlic. Saute for about 5 to 10 minutes, or until fragrant.
2. Add the broccoli, cabbage and italian seasoning. Cover and cook for 10 to 15 minutes, stirring occasionally, until the vegetables are wilted and the sausage is cooked through. Divide onto plates and enjoy!

2.9–Smoked Salmon Salad

Ingredients:
   2 Eggs
   3 cups Mixed Greens
   3 ½ ounces Smoked Salmon (sliced)
   ½ Avocado (sliced)
   2 tbsp. Avocado Oil

Sea Salt & Black Pepper (to taste)

1. Hard boil the eggs by placing them in a small pot of cold water. Bring to a boil over high heat. Once boiling, remove them from heat. Cover and let stand for 12 minutes. Transfer to a bowl of ice water to cool. Once cool, peel and slice into halves.
2. Combine all ingredients into a large bowl and toss gently before serving. Enjoy!

2.10-Roasted Chicken with Zucchini and Olives
Ingredients:

10 ½ ounces Chicken Leg, Boneless with Skin
¼ tsp. Sea Salt
2 Zucchini (medium, sliced)
1 cup Green Olives (sliced)
1 Lemon (juiced)
3 tbsp. Extra Virgin Olive Oil

1. Preheat the oven to 375F (191C).
2. Lay chicken in a large cast iron skillet, or baking sheet, and season with sea salt. Place the sliced zucchini around the chicken and top with olives, lemon juice, and olive oil.
3. Bake for 45 minutes, then broil on low for 10-15 more minutes until the top is browned. Baste with juices throughout cooking.
4. Remove from the oven and let stand for 15 minutes before serving. Enjoy!

2.11-Cauliflower Shepards Pie

Ingredients:

½ head Cauliflower (chopped into florets)

½ Yellow Onion (diced)

1 tbsp. Extra Virgin Olive Oil

1 Garlic (clove, minced)

8 ounces Extra Lean Ground Turkey

1 ½ cup Mushrooms (sliced)

1 Carrot (diced)

1 stalk Celery (diced)

1 ½ tsp. Italian Seasoning

1/8 tsp. Sea Salt

1. Preheat the oven to 350F (177C).
2. Place cauliflower florets in a medium sized saucepan, cover with water and bring to a boil. Let the florets boil until they are soft, about 15 minutes.
3. While the cauliflower is boiling, heat half of the olive oil in a large frying pan over medium heat. Add the onions and garlic, cook for 5 minutes or until onions are translucent.
4. Add the meat, and cook until browned.
5. Add the mushrooms, carrots, celery, Italian seasoning, and salt. Continue to cook for a few minutes, until the meat is cooked through. Remove from heat.
6. Drain the cauliflower and discard cooking water. Return the cauliflower to the pot and add the other half of the olive oil and a sprinkle of salt. Mash well until the cauliflower becomes almost like a puree.
7. Transfer the meat mixture to a casserole or

pie dish and distribute into an even layer. Top with the cauliflower mash and spread it evenly across the top.

8. Place in the oven and bake for 20 minutes. Turn the oven to a low broil and broil for 10 minutes or until golden. Remove from the oven and serve. Enjoy!

Acknowledgements

I want to acknowledge my parents, who do more for me than I could ever describe in words. I feel like I've hit the parent jackpot when it comes to their love and support. Mom, I inherited your passion for healing, and Dad your strong work ethic and determination. You both have always encouraged me to "think outside the box" and push myself to grow as a person and practitioner. I am so grateful for everything, especially your support. Oma daycare, clinic crew, chefs plate, the list goes on. You both demonstrate the qualities I want to show my daughters: be caring, have drive, show strength and passion for helping others.

Marco, the love of my life, and partner in crime! Your support and patience throughout this wild ride has not gone unrecognized! Thank you for your patience, and staying married to me even while I've been married to my computer during this time - I am so grateful to have a loving husband who grounds me and also lifts me up. You are an incredible dad, and husband, I love our wild life together and wouldn't want it any other way – except it being on a beach!

I am so grateful for each one of my girlfriends; all so unique and special to me. You all remind me daily to not take life so seriously. Our heart to hearts and complete ridiculousness were helpful when processing the stress of writing this book, and life! A special acknowledgement to my highschool friend who without any hesitation helped bring this book to life, and who I will cherish forever!

Most importantly, I need to acknowledge all the patients who put their trust into me, and had faith in the process. Each one of you and your families, who have become so close to me, my family and clinic and have come along with me throughout this process, each have a special place in my heart. You all have reinforced the big "why" when thinking about writing a book. It is because of all of you that I am able to help others by getting all of this powerful information out into the world.

About the Author

Lori Bouchard is an author, an entrepreneur, and licensed Naturopathic Doctor. Inspired by her mother's vibrancy and knowledge in natural medicines, she knew from a young age she would enter the healthcare field. She completed her Degree in Health Science at Western University prior to completing her Doctorate in Naturopathic Medicine, a four-year-full full-time program at the prestigious Canadian College of Naturopathic Medicine in Toronto, Ontario.

She is the owner of Oakville, Ontarios most innovative naturopathic healing centre, Inside Health Clinic, which has been helping men and women reverse complex conditions such as lyme, chronic infections, auto-immune conditions and cancer for over a decade.

She is registered through the College of Naturopathic Doctors Ontario (CONO), as well as a member of the Ontario Association of Naturopathic Doctors (OAND), Canadian Association of Naturopathic Doctors (CAND), and the Oncology

Association of Naturopathic Physicians (OncANP)

When Lori is not immersed in clinic life, she loves spending every minute with her loving husband, three beautiful daughters and handsome standard poodle who light up her life with joy each day.

Thank You

I want to say thank you to all the amazing people who have come into my life – all the warriors, rock stars and heroes who set their own rules and never accepted their diagnosis. Everyone who takes care of their own health inspires me more and more each day. I used to fear cancer, but the strength it brings out in all of you blows my mind, and it keeps me fighting and working harder every day.

Thank you so much for reading my book. As a way of saying thank you, I'd love to offer you a free class on how to live longer and stronger with breast cancer and get back to spending more time with your loved ones.

To get your copy, go to www.DrLori.ca

Bibliography

Chapter 3: Step 1- Thinking like a Cancer Survivor

(1)Andersen, B. L., Thornton, L. M., Shapiro, C. L., & et al. (2010, June 15). Biobehavioral, immune, and health benefits following recurrence for psychological intervention participants. Retrieved from https://www.ncbi.nlm.nih.gov/pmc/articles/PMC2910547/

(2) Matsunaga, M., Isowa, T., Kimura, K., Miyakoshi, M., & et al. (2008). Associations among central nervous, endocrine, and immune activities when positive emotions are elicited by looking at a favorite person. Brain, Behavior, and Immunity, 22(3), 408–417. doi: 10.1016/j.bbi.2007.09.008

(3)Brod, S., Rattazzi, L., Piras, G., & D'Acquisto, F. (2014, November). 'As above, so below' examining the interplay between emotion and the immune system. Retrieved from https://www.ncbi.nlm.nih.gov/pmc/articles/PMC4212945/ Immunology

(4)Berk, L., Calvacanti, P., Rekapalli, N., Pawar, P., & et al. (2013). EEG power spectral density activity (1-40hz) during humor associated mirthful laughter eustress compared to a stress activity: The power of gamma. PsycEXTRA Dataset. doi: 10.1037/e546872013-159

Chapter 3: Step 2-Understanding the Body to keep it Healthy

(1)Li, Y., Li, S., Zhou, Y., Meng, X., & et al. (2017, June 13). Melatonin for the prevention and treatment of cancer. Retrieved from https://www.ncbi.nlm.nih.gov/pmc/articles/PMC5503661/

(2)Jensen, K., Schauch, M., & Daniluk, J. (2015). The Adrenal Stress Connection. Coquitlam, BC: Mind Publishing.

Chapter 3: Step 3- Understanding Why Cancer Grows

(1) Liberti, M. V., & Locasale, J. W. (2016). Correction to: 'The Warburg Effect: How Does it Benefit Cancer Cells?' Trends in Biochemical Sciences, 41(3), 287. doi: 10.1016/j.tibs.2016.01.004

(2) Vyas, S., Zaganjor, E., & Haigis, M. C. (2016, July 28). Mitochondria and Cancer. Retrieved from https://www.ncbi.nlm.nih.gov/pmc/articles/PMC5036969/

(3) Zolkipli-Cunningham, Z., & Falk, M. J. (2017). Clinical effects of chemical exposures on mitochondrial function. Toxicology, 391, 90–99. doi: 10.1016/j.tox.2017.07.009

(4) Kanwal, R., & Gupta, S. (2010, August). Epigenetics and cancer. Retrieved from https://www.ncbi.nlm.nih.gov/pmc/articles/PMC2928601/#B18

(5) The Genetics of Cancer. (n.d.). Retrieved from https://www.cancer.gov/about-cancer/causes-prevention/genetics

(6) Herceg, Z., Ghantous, A., & Wild, C. P. et al. (2018, March 1). Roadmap for investigating epigenome deregulation and environmental origins of cancer. Retrieved from https://www.ncbi.nlm.nih.gov/pmc/articles/PMC6027626/

(7) Clinical Genetics of Cancer 2017: Szczecin, Poland. 21-22 September 2017. (2018, February 28). Retrieved from https://www.ncbi.nlm.nih.gov/pmc/articles/PMC5841194/

(8) McKinney, N. (2016). Naturopathic oncology: an encyclopedic guide for patients & physicians. Vancouver: Liaison Press.

(9) Buchholz, T. A., & Weil, M. M. et al. (1999). Tumor suppressor genes and breast cancer. Retrieved March 9, 2020, from https://www.ncbi.nlm.nih.gov/pubmed/10333246

(10) Holtrich, & Kourtis, K. et al. (2018, October 22). Methylation of estrogen receptor β promoter correlates with loss of ER-β expression in mammary carcinoma and is an early indication marker in premalignant lesions in: Endocrine-Related Cancer Volume 12 Issue 4 (2005). Retrieved 2019, from https://erc.bioscientifica.com/view/journals/erc/12/4/0120903.xml

(11)Brown, R. (2011). Discovering your True Balance with bioidentical hormones. Charleston, SC: Advantage.

(12)Organic Excellence. (n.d.). Xenoestrogens and How to Minimize Your Exposure. Retrieved from https://www.organicexcellence.com/blogs/news/xenoestrogens-and-how-to-minimize-your-exposure

(13)Ibid

(14)Orgel, E., & Mittelman, S. D. (2013, April). The links between insulin resistance, diabetes, and cancer. Retrieved from https://www.ncbi.nlm.nih.gov/pmc/articles/PMC3595327/

(15)McKinney, N. (2016). Naturopathic oncology: an encyclopedic guide for patients & physicians. Vancouver: Liaison Press.

(16)Laron syndrome - Genetics Home Reference - NIH. (n.d.). Retrieved from https://ghr.nlm.nih.gov/condition/laron-syndrome.

Chapter 3: Step 4– Foods that Fight Cancer

(1)Hirayama, T. (1978, June). Epidemiology of breast cancer with special reference to the role of diet. Retrieved from https://www.ncbi.nlm.nih.gov/pubmed/674105

(2)Subramani, & Ramadevi, et al. (2017, April 3). Role of Growth Hormone in Breast Cancer. Retrieved from https://academic.oup.com/endo/article/158/6/1543/3098660

(3)Campbell, T. M., & Woren, D. (2004) (2016). The China study. Ashland, OR: Blackstone Audio.

(4)Ibid

(5)Sieri, S., Agnoli, C., & Pala, V., et al. (2017, August 29). Dietary glycemic index, glycemic load, and cancer risk: results from the EPIC-Italy study. Retrieved from https://www.ncbi.nlm.nih.gov/pubmed/28851931

(6)Glycemic Index Chart: GI Ratings for Hundreds of Foods. (2019, July 1). Retrieved from https://universityhealthnews.com/daily/nutrition/glycemic-index-chart/

(7)Harvard Health Publishing. (n.d.). The lowdown on glycemic index and glycemic load. Retrieved from https://

www.health.harvard.edu/diseases-and-conditions/the-lowdown-on-glycemic-index-and-glycemic-load.

(8)Rodriguez, B. D., & Palinski-Wade, E., et al. (n.d.). The Lowdown on Glycemic Load - Diet and Nutrition Center. Retrieved from https://www.everydayhealth.com/diet-nutrition/101/nutrition-basics/the-glycemic-load.aspx

(9)Barclay, A. W., & Brand-Miller, J. C. (2005). Glycemic Index, Glycemic Load, and Glycemic Response Are Not the Same. Diabetes Care, 28(7), 1839–1840, doi: 10.2337/diacare.28.7.1839

(10)Hoffmann, C., & Dollive, S., et. al. (2013). Archaea and Fungi of the Human Gut Microbiome: Correlations with Diet and Bacterial Residents. Archaea and Fungi of the Human Gut Microbiome: Correlations with Diet and Bacterial Residents, 8(6). doi: 10.1371/journal.pone.0066019

(11)Hosseini, A., & Ghorbani, A. (2015). Cancer therapy with phytochemicals: evidence from clinical studies. Retrieved from https://www.ncbi.nlm.nih.gov/pmc/articles/PMC4418057/

(12)BreastCancer.Org. (2013, May 8). Foods Containing Phytochemicals. Retrieved from https://www.breastcancer.org/tips/nutrition/reduce_risk/foods/phytochem

(13)Stanford Health Care. (n.d.). Phytochemicals. Retrieved from https://stanfordhealthcare.org/medical-clinics/cancer-nutrition-services/reducing-cancer-risk/phytochemicals.html

(14)Hai Liu, R., & Taubes, G. (n.d.). Rui Hai Liu on Studying the Health Benefits of Whole Foods - ScienceWatch.com. Retrieved from http://archive.sciencewatch.com/inter/aut/2012/12-jan/12janLiu/

(15)Vermeulen, M., & Klöpping-Ketelaars Ineke W. A. A. (2008). Bioavailability and Kinetics of Sulforaphane in Humans after Consumption of Cooked versus Raw Broccoli. Journal of Agricultural and Food Chemistry, 56(22), 10505–10509. doi: 10.1021/jf801989e

(16)Handbook of Food Processing, Two Volume Set. (n.d.). Retrieved from https://books.google.com/books?id=aUFZDwAAQBAJ&pg=PA23&lpg=PA23&dq=journal+of

+food+chemistry+nutrition+sulforaphane&source=bl&
ots=xQ77xg-PKR&sig=ACfU3U0gSEVhDsDrkgeYxzz
rjcIG2osJ1g&hl=en

(17)Davis, E., & Kossoff, E. (2017). Fight cancer with a ketogenic diet. Cheyenne, WY: Gutsy Badger Publishing.

(18)Ibid

(19)Ziaei, S., & Halaby, R. (2017, April 7). Dietary Isoflavones and Breast Cancer Risk. Retrieved from https://www.ncbi.nlm.nih.gov/pmc/articles/PMC5590054/

(20)Pop, E. A., Fischer, L. M., & Coan, A. D. (2008). Effects of a high daily dose of soy isoflavones on DNA damage, apoptosis, and estrogenic outcomes in healthy postmenopausal women: a phase I clinical trial. Retrieved from https://www.ncbi.nlm.nih.gov/pmc/articles/PMC2574732/

(21)Fermentation: Meaning of Fermentation by Lexico. (n.d.). Retrieved from https://www.lexico.com/definition/fermentation

(22)Neustadt, J. (2020, February 26). Top Alkaline Foods to Eat & Acid Foods to Avoid. Retrieved from https://nbihealth.com/top-alkaline-foods-to-eat-acid-foods-to-avoid/

(23)Dhup, S., Dadhich, R. K., & Porporato, P. E. (2012). Multiple biological activities of lactic acid in cancer: influences on tumor growth, angiogenesis and metastasis. Retrieved from https://www.ncbi.nlm.nih.gov/pubmed/22360558

(24)Chen, L., Manautou, J. E., Rasmussen, T. P., & Zhong, X.-bo. (2019, January 15). Development of precision medicine approaches based on inter-individual variability of BCRP/ABCG2. Retrieved from https://www.sciencedirect.com/science/article/pii/S2211383518309158

(25)McDonald, J. A., Goyal, A., & Terry, M. B. (2013, September). Alcohol Intake and Breast Cancer Risk: Weighing the Overall Evidence. Retrieved from https://www.ncbi.nlm.nih.gov/pmc/articles/PMC3832299/

(26)Monroe, K. R., Stanczyk, F. Z., Besinque, K. H., & Pike, M. C. (2013). The effect of grapefruit intake on endogenous serum estrogen levels in postmenopausal women. Retrieved from https://www.ncbi.nlm.nih.gov/pmc/articles/PMC5796810/

(27)Schubert, W., Cullberg, G., Edgar, B., & Hedner, T. (2005,

April 21). Inhibition of 17β-estradiol metabolism by grapefruit juice in ovariectomized women. Retrieved from https://www.sciencedirect.com/science/article/pii/0378512294900124

(28)Monroe, K. R., Murphy, S. P., & Kolonel, L. N. (2007, August 6). Prospective study of grapefruit intake and risk of breast cancer in postmenopausal women: the Multiethnic Cohort Study. Retrieved from https://www.ncbi.nlm.nih.gov/pmc/articles/PMC2360312/

Chapter 3: Step 5–Fasting Protocols

(1)Longo, V. D., & Fontana, L. (2010). Calorie restriction and cancer prevention: metabolic and molecular mechanisms. Trends in Pharmacological Sciences, 31(2), 89–98. doi: 10.1016/j.tips.2009.11.004

(2)Marinac, C. R., Nelson, S. H., Breen, C. I., & et al. (2016, August 1). Prolonged Nightly Fasting and Breast Cancer Prognosis. Retrieved from https://www.ncbi.nlm.nih.gov/pmc/articles/PMC4982776/

(3)Can Fasting at Night Reduce Recurrence Risk? (2016, November 18). Retrieved from https://www.breastcancer.org/research-news/can-fasting-reduce-recurrence-risk

(4)Racette SB, Das SK, Bhapkar M, et al. Approaches for quantifying energy intake and calorie restriction during calorie restriction interventions in humans: the multicenter CALERIE study. American journal of physiology Endocrinology and metabolism 2012;302:E441-8.

(5)Harvie, M., Wright, C., Pegington, M., & et al. (2011). P3-09-02: Intermittent Dietary Carbohydrate Restriction Enables Weight Loss and Reduces Breast Cancer Risk Biomarkers. Poster Session Abstracts. doi: 10.1158/0008-5472.sabcs11-p3-09-02

(6)Galland, L. (2014, December). The gut microbiome and the brain. Retrieved from https://www.ncbi.nlm.nih.gov/pmc/articles/PMC4259177/

(7)Safdie, F., Brandhorst, S., Wei, M., & et al. (2012). Fasting Enhances the Response of Glioma to Chemo- and Radiotherapy. PLoS ONE, 7(9). doi: 10.1371/journal.

pone.0044603

(8)Ibid

(9)Safdie, F. M., Dorff, T., Quinn, D., & et al. (2009). Fasting and cancer treatment in humans: A case series report. Aging, 1(12), 988–1007. doi: 10.18632/aging.100114

(10)Lee, C., Raffaghello, L., Brandhorst, S., & et al. (2012). Fasting Cycles Retard Growth of Tumors and Sensitize a Range of Cancer Cell Types to Chemotherapy. Science Translational Medicine, 4(124). doi: 10.1126/scitranslmed.3003293

(11)Raffaghello, L., Safdie, F., Bianchi, G., & et al. (2010). Fasting and differential chemotherapy protection in patients. Cell Cycle, 9(22), 4474–4476. doi: 10.4161/cc.9.22.13954

Chapter 3: Step 6– How to feel Stronger through Detoxification

(1)Gennings, C., Ellis, R., & Ritter, J. K. (2012, February). Linking empirical estimates of body burden of environmental chemicals and wellness using NHANES data. Retrieved from https://www.ncbi.nlm.nih.gov/pmc/articles/PMC3249606/

(2)Centers for Disease Control and Prevention. (n.d.). Retrieved from https://www.cdc.gov/

(3)Earth / World Media Foundation / Public Radio International. (2011, April 15). Breast Cancer & Pesticides in 1991. Retrieved from http://www.loe.org/shows/segments.html?programID=11-P13-00015&segmentID=3

(4)Davis, D. L., Hoel, D., Fox, J., & et al. (1990). Annals of the New York Academy of Sciences; Volume 609 Trends in Cancer Mortality in Industrial Countries; Proceedings of the Workshop held in Capri, Italy on October 21-22, 1989, by the Collegium Ramazzini and the Municipality of Capri and the International Week of Science, October 17-25, 1989. New Yo Academy of Sciences, NY: Westin & Richter.

(5)Jensen, B. (2001). Dr. Jensen's Nature has a Remedy: Healthy

Secrets from Around the World. Los Angeles: Keats Pub.

(6) Shibata, S., Hayakawa, K., Egashira, Y., & Sanada, H. (2007, April). Hypocholesterolemic mechanism of Chlorella: Chlorella and its indigestible fraction enhance hepatic cholesterol catabolism through up-regulation of cholesterol 7alpha-hydroxylase in rats. Retrieved from https://www.ncbi.nlm.nih.gov/pubmed/17420587

(7) Barrios, J. M., & Lichtenberger, L. M. (2000, June). Role of biliary phosphatidylcholine in bile acid protection and NSAID injury of the ileal mucosa in rats. Retrieved from https://www.ncbi.nlm.nih.gov/pubmed/10833493

(8) Douglas, B. R., Jansen, J. B., Tham, R. T., & Lamers, C. B. (1990). Coffee stimulation of cholecystokinin release and gallbladder contraction in humans. The American Journal of Clinical Nutrition, 52(3), 553–556. doi: 10.1093/ajcn/52.3.553

(9) Oh, S. H., Hwang, Y. P., Choi, J. H., & et al. (2018). Kahweol inhibits proliferation and induces apoptosis by suppressing fatty acid synthase in HER2-overexpressing cancer cells. Food and Chemical Toxicology, 121, 326–335. doi: 10.1016/j.fct.2018.09.008

(10) Zhao, L., Wang, T., Dong, J., & et al. (2018, January 31). Liver-stomach disharmony pattern: theoretical basis, identification and treatment. Retrieved from https://www.sciencedirect.com/science/article/pii/S2095754818300085

(11) Hodges, R. E., & Minich, D. M. (2015). Modulation of Metabolic Detoxification Pathways Using Foods and Food-Derived Components: A Scientific Review with Clinical Application. Retrieved from https://www.ncbi.nlm.nih.gov/pmc/articles/PMC4488002/

(12) Le, J. (Last full review/revision May 2019) Content last modified May 2019. (n.d.). Drug Metabolism - Clinical Pharmacology. Retrieved from https://www.merckmanuals.com/professional/clinical-pharmacology/pharmacokinetics/drug-metabolism

(13) Ibid

(14) Vieira, C., Evangelista, S., Cirillo, R., & et al. (2000). Effect of ricinoleic acid in acute and subchronic experimental models of inflammation. Retrieved from https://www.

ncbi.nlm.nih.gov/pubmed/11200362

(15)Vieira, C., Fetzer, S., Sauer, S. K., & et al. (2001, August). Pro- and anti-inflammatory actions of ricinoleic acid: similarities and differences with capsaicin. Retrieved from https://www.ncbi.nlm.nih.gov/pubmed/11534859

(16)Hodges, R. E., & Minich, D. M. (2015). Modulation of Metabolic Detoxification Pathways Using Foods and Food-Derived Components: A Scientific Review with Clinical Application. Retrieved from https://www.ncbi. nlm.nih.gov/pmc/articles/PMC4488002/

(17)Dekhuijzen, P. N. R., & van Beurden, W. J. C. (2006). The role for N-acetylcysteine in the management of COPD. Retrieved from https://www.ncbi.nlm.nih.gov/pmc/ articles/PMC2706612/

(18)Rahman, I., & MacNee, W. (2000, September). Oxidative stress and regulation of glutathione in lung inflammation. Retrieved from https://www.ncbi.nlm.nih.gov/ pubmed/11028671

(19)Rose, S., & Fernie. (2019, October 31). All-Natural Chest Vapor Rub Recipe. Retrieved from https://gardentherapy. ca/vicks-vapo-rub-recipe/

(20)Jensen, K., Schauch, M., & Daniluk, J. (2015). The Adrenal Stress Connection. Coquitlam, BC: Mind Publishing.

(21)Ibid

Chapter 4: Additional Testing

(1)Lavine, E. (2012). Blood testing for sensitivity, allergy or intolerance to food. Canadian Medical Association Journal, 184(6), 666–668. doi: 10.1503/cmaj.110026

(2)BioTek Laboratories. (n.d.). Worldwide Leader in Specialty Medical Testing: US BioTek Laboratories. Retrieved from https://www.usbiotek.com/

(3)Advanced Hormone Testing. (n.d.). Retrieved from http:// www.Dutchtest.com

(4)Ibid

(5)GI-MAP™. (n.d.). Retrieved from https://www. designsforhealth.com/learn-more/gi-map

(6)Lee, B. K., Schwartz, B. S., Stewart, W., & Ahn, K. D. (1995,

January). Provocative chelation with DMSA and EDTA: evidence for differential access to lead storage sites. Retrieved from https://www.ncbi.nlm.nih.gov/pmc/articles/PMC1128144

(7)Aposhian, H. V., Maiorino, R. M., Rivera, M., Bruce, D. C., & et al. (1992). Human studies with the chelating agents, DMPS and DMSA. Retrieved from https://www.ncbi.nlm.nih.gov/pubmed/1331491

(8)BioTek Laboratories. (n.d.). Environmental Pollutant Profile. Retrieved from https://www.usbiotek.com/tests/environmental-pollutant-profile

(9)Toxic and Essential Elements. (n.d.). Retrieved from https://www.doctorsdata.com/toxic-essential-elements/

(10)Tongue Diagnosis in Chinese Medicine. (2020, February 19). Retrieved from https://giovanni-maciocia.com/tongue-gallery/

(11)How Molecular Iodine Attacks Breast Cancer : Oncology Times. (n.d.). Retrieved from https://journals.lww.com/oncology-times/Fulltext/2016/12250/How_Molecular_Iodine_Attacks_Breast_Cancer.13.aspx

(12)Prasad, A. S., Beck, F. W. J., Snell, D. C., & Kucuk, O. (2009). Zinc in cancer prevention. Retrieved from https://www.ncbi.nlm.nih.gov/pubmed/20155630

(13)RGCC Group. (n.d.). Retrieved from https://www.rgcc-group.com/

(14)Connealy, L. E. (2017). The cancer revolution: a groundbreaking program to reverse and prevent cancer. Boston, MA: Da Capo Life Long.

Chapter 5: Advanced Cancer Therapy

(1)Cantley, L., & Yun, J. (2020, January 20). Intravenous High-Dose Vitamin C in Cancer Therapy. Retrieved from https://www.cancer.gov/research/key-initiatives/ras/ras-central/blog/2020/yun-cantley-vitamin-c

(2)Konstat-Korzenny, E., Ascencio-Aragón, J. A., Niezen-Lugo, S., & Vázquez-López, R. (2018, February 27). Artemisinin and Its Synthetic Derivatives as a Possible Therapy for Cancer. Retrieved from https://www.ncbi.

nlm.nih.gov/pmc/articles/PMC5872176

(3)NCI Drug Dictionary. (n.d.). Retrieved from https://www. cancer.gov/publications/dictionaries/cancer-drug/def/ artesunate

(4)Bollinger, T. M. (2014). Cancer: Step Outside the Box. McKinney, TX: Infinity 510^2 Partners.

(5)Elvis, A. M., & Ekta, J. S. (2011, January). Ozone therapy: A clinical review. Retrieved from https://www.ncbi.nlm. nih.gov/pmc/articles/PMC3312702/

(6)Clavo, B., Santana-Rodríguez, N., Llontop, P., & et al. (2018, September 9). Ozone Therapy as Adjuvant for Cancer Treatment: Is Further Research Warranted? Retrieved from https://www.hindawi.com/journals/ ecam/2018/7931849/

(7)Clavo, B., Pérez, J. L., López, L., & et al. (2004, June 1). Ozone Therapy for Tumor Oxygenation: a Pilot Study. Retrieved from https://www.ncbi.nlm.nih.gov/pmc/ articles/PMC442111

(8)National Cancer Institute. (n.d.). (2019, April 25). Mistletoe Extracts (PDQ®)–Patient Version. Retrieved from https://www.cancer.gov/about-cancer/treatment/cam/ patient/mistletoe-pdq

(9)Sugarman, J. (2014, March 10). Are Mistletoe Extract Injections the Next Big Thing in Cancer Therapy? Retrieved from https://hub.jhu.edu/magazine/2014/ spring/mistletoe-therapy-cancer/

(10)Li, Y., Li, S., Zhou, Y., Meng, X., & et al. (2017, June 13). Melatonin for the prevention and treatment of cancer. Retrieved from https://www.ncbi.nlm.nih.gov/pmc/ articles/PMC5503661/

(11)González-González, A., Mediavilla, M. D., & Sánchez-Barceló, E. J. (2018, February 6). Melatonin: A Molecule for Reducing Breast Cancer Risk. Retrieved from https:// www.ncbi.nlm.nih.gov/pmc/articles/PMC6017232

(12)Pan, S. Y., Zhou, J., Gibbons, L., Canadian Cancer Registries Epidemiology Research Group [CCRERG], & et al. (2011, August 24). Antioxidants and Breast Cancer Risk- A population-based case-control study in Canada. Retrieved from https://www.ncbi.nlm.nih.gov/ pmc/articles/PMC3224257/

(13)Ibid

(14)Sun, Y., Wang, W., & Tong, Y. (2019, November 28). Berberine Inhibits Proliferative Ability of Breast Cancer Cells by Reducing Metadherin. Retrieved from https://www.ncbi.nlm.nih.gov/pubmed/31779025

(15)Yue, P., Zhang, F., Zhao, Y., & et al. (n.d.). Berberine Enhances Chemosensitivity and Induces Apoptosis Through Dose orchestrated AMPK Signaling in Breast Cancer. Retrieved from https://www.jcancer.org/v08p1679

(16)Glinsky, V. V., & Raz, A. (2009, September 28). Modified citrus pectin anti-metastatic properties: one bullet, multiple targets. Retrieved from https://www.ncbi.nlm.nih.gov/pmc/articles/PMC2782490/

(17)Jiang, J., Eliaz, I., & Sliva, D. (2013, March). Synergistic and additive effects of modified citrus pectin with two polybotanical compounds, in the suppression of invasive behavior of human breast and prostate cancer cells. Retrieved from https://www.ncbi.nlm.nih.gov/pubmed/22532035

(18)Liu, D., & Chen, Z. (2013, June). The effect of curcumin on breast cancer cells. Retrieved from https://www.ncbi.nlm.nih.gov/pmc/articles/PMC3706856/

(19)Liu, H.-T., & Ho, Y.-S. (2018, June 9). Anticancer effect of curcumin on breast cancer and stem cells. Retrieved from https://www.sciencedirect.com/science/article/pii/S2213453018300533

(20)Lockwood, K., Moesgaard, S., & Folkers, K. (1994, March 30). Partial and complete regression of breast cancer in patients in relation to dosage of coenzyme Q10. Retrieved from https://www.ncbi.nlm.nih.gov/pubmed/7908519

(21)Mathews, M. (n.d.). (2014, August). The effects of coenzyme Q10 on women with breast cancer: a systematic review protocol : JBI Evidence Synthesis. Retrieved from https://journals.lww.com/jbisrir/Fulltext/2014/12080/The_effects_of_coenzyme_Q10_on_women_with_breast.12.asp.

(22)Suzana, S., Cham, B. G., Ahmad Rohi, G., Mohd Rizal, R., & et al. (2009, March). Relationship between selenium and breast cancer: a case-control study in the Klang

Valley. Retrieved from https://www.ncbi.nlm.nih.gov/pubmed/19352569

(23)Vinceti, M., Filippini, T., Del Giovane, C., Dennert, G., & et al. (2018, January 29). Selenium for preventing cancer. Retrieved from https://www.ncbi.nlm.nih.gov/pubmed/29376219

(24)Wang, R., Yang, L., Li, S., Ye, D., & et al. (2018, January 21). Quercetin Inhibits Breast Cancer Stem Cells via Downregulation of Aldehyde Dehydrogenase 1A1 (ALDH1A1), Chemokine Receptor Type 4 (CXCR4), Mucin 1 (MUC1), and Epithelial Cell Adhesion Molecule (EpCAM). Retrieved from https://www.ncbi.nlm.nih.gov/pmc/articles/PMC5788241/

(25)Deng, X.-H., Song, H.-Y., Zhou, Y.-F., & et al. (2013, November). Effects of quercetin on the proliferation of breast cancer cells and expression of survivin in vitro. Retrieved from https://www.ncbi.nlm.nih.gov/pmc/articles/PMC3820718/

(26)Kasiri, N., Rahmati, M., Ahmadi, L. et al. Therapeutic potential of quercetin on human breast cancer in different dimensions. Inflammopharmacol 28, 39–62 (2020). https://doi.org/10.1007/s10787-019-00660-y

(27)Eliaz, I., Hotchkiss, A. T., Fishman, M. L., & Rode, D. (2006, October). The effect of modified citrus pectin on urinary excretion of toxic elements. Retrieved from https://www.ncbi.nlm.nih.gov/pubmed/16835878

(28)Crinnion, W. J. (2008, November 4). Alternative Medicine Review. Is Modified Citrus Pectin an Effective Mobilizer of Heavy Metals in Humans. Retrieved from http://www.altmedrev.com/archive/publications/13/4/283.pdf

(29)University of Salford. (2017, March 8). Vitamin C is effective in targeting cancer stem cells. Retrieved from https://www.sciencedaily.com/releases/2017/03/170308083940.htm

(30)Fiorillo, M., Tóth, F., Sotgia, F., & Lisanti, M. P. (2019, April 19). Doxycycline, Azithromycin and Vitamin C (DAV): A potent combination therapy for targeting mitochondria and eradicating cancer stem cells (CSCs). Retrieved from https://www.ncbi.nlm.nih.gov/pmc/articles/PMC6520007/

(31)Fiorillo, M., Tóth, F., Sotgia, F., & Lisanti, M. P. (2019,

April 19). Doxycycline, Azithromycin and Vitamin C (DAV): A potent combination therapy for targeting mitochondria and eradicating cancer stem cells (CSCs). Retrieved from https://www.ncbi.nlm.nih.gov/pmc/articles/PMC6520007/

(32)Ginestier, C., Wicinski, J., Cervera, N., Monville, F., & et al. (2009, October 15). Retinoid signaling regulates breast cancer stem cell differentiation. Retrieved from https://www.ncbi.nlm.nih.gov/pubmed/19806016

(33)University of Salford. (2017, March 8). Vitamin C is effective in targeting cancer stem cells. Retrieved from https://www.sciencedaily.com/releases/2017/03/170308083940.htm

(34)Koçak, N., Nergiz, S., Yıldırım, İ. H., & Duran, Y. (2018, September 30). Vitamin D can be used as a supplement against cancer stem cells. Retrieved from https://www.ncbi.nlm.nih.gov/pubmed/30301502

(35) Lin, P.-H., Sermersheim, M., Li, H., & et al. (2017, December 24). Zinc in Wound Healing Modulation. Retrieved from https://www.ncbi.nlm.nih.gov/pmc/articles/PMC5793244/

(36)Ebaid, H., Salem, A., Sayed, A., & Metwalli, A. (2011, December 14). Whey protein enhances normal inflammatory responses during cutaneous wound healing in diabetic rats. Retrieved from https://www.ncbi.nlm.nih.gov/pmc/articles/PMC3254143/

(37)Lei, Z., Cao, Z., Yang, Z., & et al. (2019, May). Rosehip Oil Promotes Excisional Wound Healing by Accelerating the Phenotypic Transition of Macrophages. Retrieved from https://www.ncbi.nlm.nih.gov/pubmed/30199901

(38)Kim, H. H., Kawazoe, T., Han, D.-W., & et al. (2008). Enhanced wound healing by an epigallocatechin gallate-incorporated collagen sponge in diabetic mice. Retrieved from https://www.ncbi.nlm.nih.gov/pubmed/19128267

(39)Musalmah, M., Nizrana, M. Y., Fairuz, A. H., & et al. (2005, June). Comparative effects of palm vitamin E and alpha-tocopherol on healing and wound tissue antioxidant enzyme levels in diabetic rats. Retrieved from https://www.ncbi.nlm.nih.gov/pubmed/16149736

(40) Lin, P.-H., Sermersheim, M., Li, H., & et al. (2017, December 24). Zinc in Wound Healing Modulation.

Retrieved from https://www.ncbi.nlm.nih.gov/pmc/articles/PMC5793244/

(41)University of Salford. (2017, March 8). Vitamin C is effective in targeting cancer stem cells. Retrieved from https://www.sciencedaily.com/releases/2017/03/170308083940.htm

(42)Stavrou, G., & Kotzampassi, K. (2017). Gut microbiome, surgical complications and probiotics. Retrieved from https://www.ncbi.nlm.nih.gov/pmc/articles/PMC5198246/

(43)Soheilifar, S., Bidgoli, M., Hooshyarfard, A., & et al. (2018, September). Effect of Oral Bromelain on Wound Healing, Pain, and Bleeding at Donor Site Following Free Gingival Grafting: A Clinical Trial. Retrieved from https://www.ncbi.nlm.nih.gov/pmc/articles/PMC6397736/

(44)McDaniel, J. C., Belury, M., Ahijevych, K., & Blakely, W. (2008). Omega-3 fatty acids effect on wound healing. Retrieved from https://www.ncbi.nlm.nih.gov/pubmed/18471252

(45)Menéndez-Menéndez, J., & Martínez-Campa, C. (2018, October 2). Melatonin: An Anti-Tumor Agent in Hormone-Dependent Cancers. Retrieved from https://www.ncbi.nlm.nih.gov/pmc/articles/PMC6189685/

(46)Marvibaigi, M., Supriyanto, E., Amini, N., & et al. (2014). Preclinical and clinical effects of mistletoe against breast cancer. Retrieved from https://www.ncbi.nlm.nih.gov/pmc/articles/PMC4127267/

(47)Zhou, R., Chen, H., Chen, J., & et al. (2018, March 9). Extract from Astragalus membranaceus inhibit breast cancer cells proliferation via PI3K/AKT/mTOR signaling pathway. Retrieved from https://www.ncbi.nlm.nih.gov/pubmed/29523109

(48)Suárez-Arroyo, I. J., Loperena-Alvarez, Y., Rosario-Acevedo, R., & Martínez-Montemayor, M. M. (2017, March). A Promising Adjuvant Treatment for Breast Cancer. Retrieved from https://www.ncbi.nlm.nih.gov/pmc/articles/PMC5533290/

(49)Choi, S. W. (1999, August). Vitamin B12 deficiency: a new risk factor for breast cancer? Retrieved from https://www.ncbi.nlm.nih.gov/pubmed/10518411

(50)Farhood, B., Goradel, N. H., Mortezaee, K., & et al. (2019,

March). Melatonin as an adjuvant in radiotherapy for radioprotection and radiosensitization. Retrieved from https://www.ncbi.nlm.nih.gov/pubmed/30136132

(51)Hardman, W. E., Sun, L. Z., Short, N., & Cameron, I. L. (2005, April 28). Dietary omega-3 fatty acids and ionizing irradiation on human breast cancer xenograft growth and angiogenesis. Retrieved from https://www.ncbi.nlm.nih.gov/pmc/articles/PMC1097743/

(52)Wang, J., Liu, Q., & Yang, Q. (2012, November). Radiosensitization effects of berberine on human breast cancer cells. Retrieved from https://www.ncbi.nlm.nih.gov/pubmed/22895634

(53)Di Franco, R., Calvanese, M. G., Murino, P., & et al. (2012, January 30). Skin toxicity from external beam radiation therapy in breast cancer patients: protective effects of Resveratrol, Lycopene, Vitamin C and anthocianin (Ixor®). Retrieved from https://www.ncbi.nlm.nih.gov/pmc/articles/PMC3283474/

(54)Verma, P., Jahan, S., Kim, T. H., & Goyal, P. K. (2011, September). Management of Radiation Injuries by Panax ginseng Extract. Retrieved from https://www.ncbi.nlm.nih.gov/pmc/articles/PMC3659536/

(55) Lu, S., Ke, Y., Wu, C. et al. Radiosensitization of clioquinol and zinc in human cancer cell lines. BMC Cancer 18, 448 (2018). https://doi.org/10.1186/s12885-018-4264-2

(56)Breast Cancer Organization. (2020, March 28). Tamoxifen: Uses, Side Effects, and More. Retrieved from https://www.breastcancer.org/treatment/hormonal/serms/tamoxifen

(57)Breast Cancer Organization. (2019, March 15). Heart Problems Caused by Herceptin May Be More Common Than Thought. Retrieved from https://www.breastcancer.org/research-news/20111208b

(58)Wang, J., Xiong, X., & Feng, B. (2013). Effect of crataegus usage in cardiovascular disease prevention: an evidence-based approach. Retrieved from https://www.ncbi.nlm.nih.gov/pmc/articles/PMC3891531/

(59)Ghasemian, M., Owlia, S., & Owlia, M. B. (2016). Review of Anti-Inflammatory Herbal Medicines. Retrieved from https://www.ncbi.nlm.nih.gov/pmc/articles/

324

PMC4877453/

(60)Meyers, B. A. (2014). Pemf - the fifth element of health: learn why pulsed electromagnetic field therapy (Pemf) supercharges your health like nothing else! Bloomington, IN: Balboa Press, a division of Hay House.

Recipe Index

(1)That Clean Life: Simple Personalized Nutrition Software for Health Professionals. Retrieved from https://thatcleanlife.com/

References

Advanced Hormone Testing. (n.d.). Retrieved from http://www.Dutchtest.com/

Aposhian, H. V., Maiorino, R. M., Rivera, M., Bruce, D. C., & et al. (1992). Human studies with the chelating agents, DMPS and DMSA. Retrieved from https://www.ncbi.nlm.nih.gov/pubmed/1331491

Barclay, A. W., & Brand-Miller, J. C. (2005). Glycemic Index, Glycemic Load, and Glycemic Response Are Not the Same. Diabetes Care, 28(7), 1839–1840. doi: 10.2337/diacare.28.7.1839

Barrios, J. M., & Lichtenberger, L. M. (2000, June). Role of biliary phosphatidylcholine in bile acid protection and NSAID injury of the ileal mucosa in rats. Retrieved from https://www.ncbi.nlm.nih.gov/pubmed/10833493

Berk, L., Calvacanti, P., Rekapalli, N., Pawar, P., & et al. (2013). EEG power spectral density activity (1-40hz) during humor associated mirthful laughter eustress compared to a stress activity: The power of gamma. PsycEXTRA Dataset. doi: 10.1037/e546872013-159

BioTek Laboratories. (n.d.). Worldwide Leader in Specialty Medical Testing: US BioTek Laboratories. Retrieved from https://www.usbiotek.com/

BioTek Laboratories. (n.d.). Environmental Pollutant Profile. Retrieved from https://www.usbiotek.com/tests/environmental-pollutant-profile

Bollinger, T. M. (2014). Cancer: step outside the box. McKinney, TX: Infinity 510² Partners.

Breast Cancer Organization. (2019, March 15). Heart Problems Caused by Herceptin May Be More Common Than

Thought. Retrieved from https://www.breastcancer.org/research-news/20111208b

Breast Cancer Organization. (2020, March 28). Tamoxifen: Uses, Side Effects, and More. Retrieved from https://www.breastcancer.org/treatment/hormonal/serms/tamoxifen

BreastCancer.Org. (2015, February 5). Foods Containing Phytochemicals. Retrieved from https://www.breastcancer.org/tips/nutrition/reduce_risk/foods/phytochem

Brod, S., Rattazzi, L., Piras, G., & D'Acquisto, F. (2014, November). 'As above, so below' examining the interplay between emotion and the immune system. Retrieved from https://www.ncbi.nlm.nih.gov/pmc/articles/PMC4212945/ Immunology

Brown, R. (2011). Discovering your Truebalance with bioidentical hormones. Charleston, SC: Advantage.

Buchholz, T. A., & Weil, M. M. (1999). Tumor suppressor genes and breast cancer. Retrieved March 9, 2020, from https://www.ncbi.nlm.nih.gov/pubmed/10333246

Cameron, E., & Pauling, L. (2018). Cancer and vitamin C: a discussion of the nature, causes, prevention, and treatment of cancer with special reference to the value of vitamin C. Philadelphia: Camino Books, Inc.

Campbell, T. M., & Woren, D. (2016). The China study. Ashland, OR: Blackstone Audio.

Can Fasting at Night Reduce Recurrence Risk? (2016, November 18). Retrieved from https://www.breastcancer.org/research-news/can-fasting-reduce-recurrence-risk

Cantley, L., & Yun, J. (2020, January 20). Intravenous High-Dose Vitamin C in Cancer Therapy. Retrieved from https://www.cancer.gov/research/key-initiatives/ras/ras-central/blog/2020/yun-cantley-vitamin-c

Centers for Disease Control and Prevention. (n.d.). Retrieved from https://www.cdc.gov/

Chen, L., Manautou, J. E., Rasmussen, T. P., & Zhong, X.-bo. (2019, January 15). Development of precision medicine approaches based on inter-individual variability of BCRP/ABCG2. Retrieved from https://www.sciencedirect.com/science/article/pii/S2211383518309158

Cheng, C.-W., Adams, G. B., Perin, L., Wei, M., & et al. (2016). Prolonged Fasting Reduces IGF-1/PKA to Promote Hematopoietic-Stem-Cell-Based Regeneration and Reverse Immunosuppression. Cell Stem Cell, 18(2), 291–292. doi: 10.1016/j.stem.2016.01.018

Choi, S. W. (1999, August). Vitamin B12 deficiency: a new risk factor for breast cancer? Retrieved from https://www.ncbi.nlm.nih.gov/pubmed/10518411

Clavo, B., Pérez, J. L., López, L., & et al. (2004, June 1). Ozone Therapy for Tumor Oxygenation: a Pilot Study. Retrieved from https://www.ncbi.nlm.nih.gov/pmc/articles/PMC442111

Clavo, B., Santana-Rodríguez, N., Llontop, P., & et al. (2018, September 9). Ozone Therapy as Adjuvant for Cancer Treatment: Is Further Research Warranted? Retrieved from https://www.hindawi.com/journals/ecam/2018/7931849/

Clinical Genetics of Cancer 2017: Szczecin, Poland. 21-22 September 2017. (2018, February 28). Retrieved from https://www.ncbi.nlm.nih.gov/pmc/articles/PMC5841194/

Colman, R. J., Anderson, R. M., Johnson, S. C., Kastman, E. K., & et al. (2009). Caloric Restriction Delays Disease Onset and Mortality in Rhesus Monkeys. Science, 325(5937), 201–204. doi: 10.1126/science.1173635

Connealy, L. E. (2017). The cancer revolution: a groundbreaking program to rerverse and prevent cancer. Boston, MA: Da Capo Life Long.

Crinnion, W. J. (2008, November 4). Alternative Medicine Review. Alternative Medicine Review. Retrieved from http://www.altmedrev.com/archive/publications/13/4/283.pdf

Davis, D. L., Hoel, D., Fox, J., & et al. (1990). Annals of the New York Academy of Sciences; Volume 609 Trends in Cancer Mortality in Industrial Countries; Proceedings of the Workshop held in Capri, Italy on October 21-22, 1989, by the Collegium Ramazzini and the Municipality of Capri and the International Week of Science, October 17-25, 1989. New Yo Academy of Sciences, NY: Westin & Richter.

Davis, E., & Kossoff, E. (2017). Fight cancer with a ketogenic diet. Cheyenne, WY: Gutsy Badger Publishing.

Dekhuijzen, P. N. R., & van Beurden, W. J. C. (2006). The role for N-acetylcysteine in the management of COPD. Retrieved from https://www.ncbi.nlm.nih.gov/pmc/articles/PMC2706612/

Deng, X.-H., Song, H.-Y., Zhou, Y.-F., & et al. (2013, November). Effects of quercetin on the proliferation of breast cancer cells and expression of survivin in vitro. Retrieved from https://www.ncbi.nlm.nih.gov/pmc/articles/PMC3820718/

Dhup, S., Dadhich, R. K., & Porporato, P. E. (2012). Multiple biological activities of lactic acid in cancer: influences on tumor growth, angiogenesis and metastasis. Retrieved from https://www.ncbi.nlm.nih.gov/pubmed/22360558

Di Franco, R., Calvanese, M. G., Murino, P., & et al. (2012, January 30). Skin toxicity from external beam radiation therapy in breast cancer patients: protective effects of Resveratrol, Lycopene, Vitamin C and anthocianin (Ixor®). Retrieved from https://www.ncbi.nlm.nih.gov/pmc/articles/PMC3283474/

Douglas, B. R., Jansen, J. B., Tham, R. T., & Lamers, C. B. (1990). Coffee stimulation of cholecystokinin release and gallbladder contraction in humans. The American Journal of Clinical Nutrition, 52(3), 553–556. doi: 10.1093/ajcn/52.3.553

Earth / World Media Foundation / Public Radio International. (2011, April 15). Breast Cancer & Pesticides in 1991. Retrieved from http://www.loe.org/shows/segments.html?programID=11-P13-00015&segmentID=3

Ebaid, H., Salem, A., Sayed, A., & Metwalli, A. (2011, December 14). Whey protein enhances normal inflammatory responses during cutaneous wound healing in diabetic rats. Retrieved from https://www.ncbi.nlm.nih.gov/pmc/articles/PMC3254143/

Eliaz, I., Hotchkiss, A. T., Fishman, M. L., & Rode, D. (2006, October). The effect of modified citrus pectin on urinary excretion of toxic elements. Retrieved from https://www.ncbi.nlm.nih.gov/pubmed/16835878

Elvis, A. M., & Ekta, J. S. (2011, January). Ozone therapy: A clinical review. Retrieved from https://www.ncbi.nlm.nih.gov/pmc/articles/PMC3312702/

Farhood, B., Goradel, N. H., Mortezaee, K., & et al. (2019, March). Melatonin as an adjuvant in radiotherapy for radioprotection and radiosensitization. Retrieved from https://www.ncbi.nlm.nih.gov/pubmed/30136132

Fermentation: Meaning of Fermentation by Lexico. (n.d.). Retrieved from https://www.lexico.com/definition/

fermentation

Fiorillo, M., Tóth, F., Sotgia, F., & Lisanti, M. P. (2019, April 19). Doxycycline, Azithromycin and Vitamin C (DAV): A potent combination therapy for targeting mitochondria and eradicating cancer stem cells (CSCs). Retrieved from https://www.ncbi.nlm.nih.gov/pmc/articles/PMC6520007/

Galland, L. (2014, December). The gut microbiome and the brain. Retrieved from https://www.ncbi.nlm.nih.gov/pmc/articles/PMC4259177/

Gennings, C., Ellis, R., & Ritter, J. K. (2012, February). Linking empirical estimates of body burden of environmental chemicals and wellness using NHANES data. Retrieved from https://www.ncbi.nlm.nih.gov/pmc/articles/PMC3249606/

Ghasemian, M., Owlia, S., & Owlia, M. B. (2016). Review of Anti-Inflammatory Herbal Medicines. Retrieved from https://www.ncbi.nlm.nih.gov/pmc/articles/PMC4877453/

GI-MAP™ .(n.d.). Retrieved from https://www.designsforhealth.com/learn-more/gi-map

Ginestier, C., Wicinski, J., Cervera, N., Monville, F., & et al. (2009, October 15). Retinoid signaling regulates breast cancer stem cell differentiation. Retrieved from https://www.ncbi.nlm.nih.gov/pubmed/19806016

Ginestier, C., Wicinski, J., Cervera, N., Monville, F., & et al. (2009, October 15). Retinoid signaling regulates breast cancer stem cell differentiation. Retrieved from https://www.ncbi.nlm.nih.gov/pmc/articles/PMC2861502

Glinsky, V. V., & Raz, A. (2009, September 28). Modified citrus pectin anti-metastatic properties: one bullet, multiple targets. Retrieved from https://www.ncbi.nlm.nih.gov/

pmc/articles/PMC2782490/

Glycemic Index Chart: GI Ratings for Hundreds of Foods. (2019, July 1). Retrieved from https://universityhealthnews. com/daily/nutrition/glycemic-index-chart/

González-González, A., Mediavilla, M. D., & Sánchez-Barceló, E. J. (2018, February 6). Melatonin: A Molecule for Reducing Breast Cancer Risk. Retrieved from https:// www.ncbi.nlm.nih.gov/pmc/articles/PMC6017232

Hai Liu, R., & Taubes, G. (n.d.). Rui Hai Liu on Studying the Health Benefits of Whole Foods - ScienceWatch.com. Retrieved from http://archive.sciencewatch.com/inter/ aut/2012/12-jan/12janLiu/

Handbook of Food Processing, Two Volume Set. (n.d.). Retrieved from https://books.google.com/books?id=aU FZDwAAQBAJ&pg=PA23&lpg=PA23&dq=journal+of +food+chemistry+nutrition+sulforaphane&source=bl& ots=xQ77xg-PKR&sig=ACfU3U0gSEVhDsDrkgeYxzz rjcIG2osJ1g&hl=en

Hardman, W. E., Sun, L. Z., Short, N., & Cameron, I. L. (2005, April 28). Dietary omega-3 fatty acids and ionizing irradiation on human breast cancer xenograft growth and angiogenesis. Retrieved from https://www.ncbi.nlm.nih. gov/pmc/articles/PMC1097743/

Harvard Health Publishing. (n.d.). The lowdown on glycemic index and glycemic load. Retrieved from https:// www.health.harvard.edu/diseases-and-conditions/the-lowdown-on-glycemic-index-and-glycemic-load

Harvie, M., Wright, C., Pegington, M., & et al. (2011). P3-09-02: Intermittent Dietary Carbohydrate Restriction Enables Weight Loss and Reduces Breast Cancer Risk Biomarkers. Poster Session Abstracts. doi: 10.1158/0008-5472.sabcs11-p3-09-02

Herceg, Z., Ghantous, A., & Wild, C. P. (2018, March 1). Roadmap for investigating epigenome deregulation and environmental origins of cancer. Retrieved from https://www.ncbi.nlm.nih.gov/pmc/articles/PMC6027626/

Hirayama, T. (1978, June). Epidemiology of breast cancer with special reference to the role of diet. Retrieved from https://www.ncbi.nlm.nih.gov/pubmed/674105

Hodges, R. E., & Minich, D. M. (2015). Modulation of Metabolic Detoxification Pathways Using Foods and Food-Derived Components: A Scientific Review with Clinical Application. Retrieved from https://www.ncbi.nlm.nih.gov/pmc/articles/PMC4488002/

Hoffmann, C., & Dollive, S. (2013). Archaea and Fungi of the Human Gut Microbiome: Correlations with Diet and Bacterial Residents. Archaea and Fungi of the Human Gut Microbiome: Correlations with Diet and Bacterial Residents, 8(6). doi: 10.1371/journal.pone.0066019

Holtrich, & Kourtis, K. (2018, October 22). Methylation of estrogen receptor β promoter correlates with loss of ER-β expression in mammary carcinoma and is an early indication marker in premalignant lesions in: Endocrine-Related Cancer Volume 12 Issue 4 (2005). Retrieved 2019, from https://erc.bioscientifica.com/view/journals/erc/12/4/0120903.xml

Hosseini, A., & Ghorbani, A. (2015). Cancer therapy with phytochemicals: evidence from clinical studies. Retrieved from https://www.ncbi.nlm.nih.gov/pmc/articles/PMC4418057/

How Molecular Iodine Attacks Breast Cancer : Oncology Times. (n.d.). Retrieved from https://journals.lww.com/oncology-times/Fulltext/2016/12250/How_Molecular_Iodine_Attacks_Breast_Cancer.13.aspx

Jensen, B., & Bell, S. (1981). Tissue cleansing through bowel management: from the simple to the ultimate. Escondido, CA: Bernard Jensen.

Jensen, B. (2000). Dr. Jensen's Juicing Therapy: Nature's Way to Better Health and a Longer Life. New York: McGraw-Hill.

Jensen, B. (2001). Dr. Jensen's nature has a remedy: healthy secrets from around the world. Los Angeles: Keats Pub.

Jensen, B. (2002). Dr. Jensen's Guide to Body Chemistry & Nutrition. New Delhi: Viva Books.

Jensen, K., Schauch, M., & Daniluk, J. (2015). The Adrenal Stress Connection. Coquitlam, BC: Mind Publishing.

Jiang, J., Eliaz, I., & Sliva, D. (2013, March). Synergistic and additive effects of modified citrus pectin with two polybotanical compounds, in the suppression of invasive behavior of human breast and prostate cancer cells. Retrieved from https://www.ncbi.nlm.nih.gov/pubmed/22532035

K, M., J, W., I, S., & A, H. (2015). Glycemic Index and Glycemic Load of a Carbohydrate-Rich and Protein-Rich Formula Diet. Journal of Nutrition and Health Sciences, 2(4). doi: 10.15744/2393-9060.2.404

Kalaany, N. Y., & Sabatini, D. M. (2009). Tumours with PI3K activation are resistant to dietary restriction. Nature, 458(7239), 725–731. doi: 10.1038/nature07782

Kanwal, R., & Gupta, S. (2010, August). Epigenetics and cancer. Retrieved from https://www.ncbi.nlm.nih.gov/pmc/articles/PMC2928601/#B18

Kasiri, N., Rahmati, M., Ahmadi, L. et al. Therapeutic potential of quercetin on human breast cancer in different dimensions. Inflammopharmacol 28, 39–62 (2020). https://doi.org/10.1007/s10787-019-00660-y

334

Kim, H. H., Kawazoe, T., Han, D.-W., & et al. (2008). Enhanced wound healing by an epigallocatechin gallate-incorporated collagen sponge in diabetic mice. Retrieved from https://www.ncbi.nlm.nih.gov/pubmed/19128267

Konstat-Korzenny, E., Ascencio-Aragón, J. A., Niezen-Lugo, S., & Vázquez-López, R. (2018, February 27). Artemisinin and Its Synthetic Derivatives as a Possible Therapy for Cancer. Retrieved from https://www.ncbi.nlm.nih.gov/pmc/articles/PMC5872176

Koçak, N., Nergiz, S., Yıldırım, İ. H., & Duran, Y. (2018, September 30). Vitamin D can be used as a supplement against cancer stem cells. Retrieved from https://www.ncbi.nlm.nih.gov/pubmed/30301502

Laron syndrome - Genetics Home Reference - NIH. (n.d.). Retrieved from https://ghr.nlm.nih.gov/condition/laron-syndrome

Lavine, E. (2012). Blood testing for sensitivity, allergy or intolerance to food. Canadian Medical Association Journal, 184(6), 666–668. doi: 10.1503/cmaj.110026

Le, J., By, Le, J., & Last full review/revision May 2019| Content last modified May 2019. (n.d.). Drug Metabolism - Clinical Pharmacology. Retrieved from https://www.merckmanuals.com/professional/clinical-pharmacology/pharmacokinetics/drug-metabolism

Lee, B. K., Schwartz, B. S., Stewart, W., & Ahn, K. D. (1995, January). Provocative chelation with DMSA and EDTA: evidence for differential access to lead storage sites. Retrieved from https://www.ncbi.nlm.nih.gov/pmc/articles/PMC1128144

Lee, C., & Longo, V. D. (2011). Fasting vs dietary restriction in cellular protection and cancer treatment: from model organisms to patients. Oncogene, 30(30), 3305–3316. doi: 10.1038/onc.2011.91

Lee, C., Raffaghello, L., Brandhorst, S., & et al. (2012). Fasting Cycles Retard Growth of Tumors and Sensitize a Range of Cancer Cell Types to Chemotherapy. Science Translational Medicine, 4(124). doi: 10.1126/scitranslmed.3003293

Lei, Z., Cao, Z., Yang, Z., & et al. (2019, May). Rosehip Oil Promotes Excisional Wound Healing by Accelerating the Phenotypic Transition of Macrophages. Retrieved from https://www.ncbi.nlm.nih.gov/pubmed/30199901

Li, Y., Li, S., Zhou, Y., Meng, X., & et al. (2017, June 13). Melatonin for the prevention and treatment of cancer. Retrieved from https://www.ncbi.nlm.nih.gov/pmc/articles/PMC5503661/

Liberti, M. V., & Locasale, J. W. (2016). Correction to: 'The Warburg Effect: How Does it Benefit Cancer Cells?' Trends in Biochemical Sciences, 41(3), 287. doi: 10.1016/j.tibs.2016.01.004

Life, T. C. (n.d.). That Clean Life: Simple Personalized Nutrition Software for Health Professionals. Retrieved from https://thatcleanlife.com/

Lin, P.-H., Sermersheim, M., Li, H., & et al. (2017, December 24). Zinc in Wound Healing Modulation. Retrieved from https://www.ncbi.nlm.nih.gov/pmc/articles/PMC5793244/

Liu, D., & Chen, Z. (2013, June). The effect of curcumin on breast cancer cells. Retrieved from https://www.ncbi.nlm.nih.gov/pmc/articles/PMC3706856/

Liu, H.-T., & Ho, Y.-S. (2018, June 9). Anticancer effect of curcumin on breast cancer and stem cells. Retrieved from https://www.sciencedirect.com/science/article/pii/S2213453018300533

Lockwood, K., Moesgaard, S., & Folkers, K. (1994, March

30). Partial and complete regression of breast cancer in patients in relation to dosage of coenzyme Q10. Retrieved from https://www.ncbi.nlm.nih.gov/pubmed/7908519

Longo, V. D., & Fontana, L. (2010). Calorie restriction and cancer prevention: metabolic and molecular mechanisms. Trends in Pharmacological Sciences, 31(2), 89–98. doi: 10.1016/j.tips.2009.11.004

Lu, S., Ke, Y., Wu, C. et al. Radiosensitization of clioquinol and zinc in human cancer cell lines. BMC Cancer 18, 448 (2018). https://doi.org/10.1186/s12885-018-4264-2

Marinac, C. R., Nelson, S. H., Breen, C. I., & et al. (2016, August 1). Prolonged Nightly Fasting and Breast Cancer Prognosis. Retrieved from https://www.ncbi.nlm.nih.gov/pmc/articles/PMC4982776/

Marinac, C. R., Nelson, S. H., Breen, C. I., Hartman, S. J., & et. al. (2016). Prolonged Nightly Fasting and Breast Cancer Prognosis. JAMA Oncology, 2(8), 1049. doi: 10.1001/jamaoncol.2016.0164

Marvibaigi, M., Supriyanto, E., Amini, N., & et al. (2014). Preclinical and clinical effects of mistletoe against breast cancer. Retrieved from https://www.ncbi.nlm.nih.gov/pmc/articles/PMC4127267/

Mathews, M. (n.d.). (2014, August). The effects of coenzyme Q10 on women with breast cancer: a systematic review protocol : JBI Evidence Synthesis. Retrieved from https://journals.lww.com/jbisrir/Fulltext/2014/12080/The_effects_of_coenzyme_Q10_on_women_with_breast.12.aspx

Matsunaga, M., Isowa, T., Kimura, K., Miyakoshi, M., & et al. (2008). Associations among central nervous, endocrine, and immune activities when positive emotions are elicited by looking at a favorite person. Brain, Behavior, and Immunity, 22(3), 408–417. doi: 10.1016/j.

bbi.2007.09.008

McDaniel, J. C., Belury, M., Ahijevych, K., & Blakely, W. (2008). Omega-3 fatty acids effect on wound healing. Retrieved from https://www.ncbi.nlm.nih.gov/pubmed/18471252

McDonald, J. A., Goyal, A., & Terry, M. B. (2013, September). Alcohol Intake and Breast Cancer Risk: Weighing the Overall Evidence. Retrieved from https://www.ncbi.nlm. nih.gov/pmc/articles/PMC3832299/

McKinney, N. (2016). Naturopathic oncology: an encyclopedic guide for patients & physicians. Vancouver: Liaison Press.

Menéndez-Menéndez, J., & Martínez-Campa, C. (2018, October 2). Melatonin: An Anti-Tumor Agent in Hormone-Dependent Cancers. Retrieved from https://www.ncbi. nlm.nih.gov/pmc/articles/PMC6189685/

Meyers, B. A. (2014). Pemf - the fifth element of health: learn why pulsed electromagnetic field therapy (Pemf) supercharges your health like nothing else! Bloomington, IN: Balboa Press, a division of Hay House.

Michalsen, A., & Li, C. (2013). Fasting Therapy for Treating and Preventing Disease - Current State of Evidence. Forschende Komplementärmedizin / Research in Complementary Medicine, 20(6), 444–453. doi: 10.1159/000357765

Monroe, K. R., Murphy, S. P., & Kolonel, L. N. (2007, August 6). Prospective study of grapefruit intake and risk of breast cancer in postmenopausal women: the Multiethnic Cohort Study. Retrieved from https://www.ncbi.nlm.nih. gov/pmc/articles/PMC2360312/

Monroe, K. R., Stanczyk, F. Z., Besinque, K. H., & Pike, M. C. (2013). The effect of grapefruit intake on endogenous serum estrogen levels in postmenopausal women.

Retrieved from https://www.ncbi.nlm.nih.gov/pmc/articles/PMC5796810/

Musalmah, M., Nizrana, M. Y., Fairuz, A. H., & et al. (2005, June). Comparative effects of palm vitamin E and alpha-tocopherol on healing and wound tissue antioxidant enzyme levels in diabetic rats. Retrieved from https://www.ncbi.nlm.nih.gov/pubmed/16149736

National Cancer Institute. (n.d.). Mistletoe Extracts (PDQ®)–Patient Version. Retrieved from https://www.cancer.gov/about-cancer/treatment/cam/patient/mistletoe-pdq

NCI Drug Dictionary. (n.d.). Retrieved from https://www.cancer.gov/publications/dictionaries/cancer-drug/def/artesunate

Neustadt, J. (2020, February 26). Top Alkaline Foods to Eat & Acid Foods to Avoid. Retrieved from https://nbihealth.com/top-alkaline-foods-to-eat-acid-foods-to-avoid/

Oh, S. H., Hwang, Y. P., Choi, J. H., & et al. (2018). Kahweol inhibits proliferation and induces apoptosis by suppressing fatty acid synthase in HER2-overexpressing cancer cells. Food and Chemical Toxicology, 121, 326–335. doi: 10.1016/j.fct.2018.09.008

Ong, K. R., Sims, A. H., Harvie, M., Chapman, M., Dunn, W. B., Broadhurst, D., … Howell, A. (2009). Biomarkers of Dietary Energy Restriction in Women at Increased Risk of Breast Cancer. Cancer Prevention Research, 2(8), 720–731. doi: 10.1158/1940-6207.capr-09-0008

Organic Excellence. (n.d.). Xenoestrogens and How to Minimize Your Exposure. Retrieved from https://www.organicexcellence.com/blogs/news/xenoestrogens-and-how-to-minimize-your-exposure

Orgel, E., & Mittelman, S. D. (2013, April). The links between insulin resistance, diabetes, and cancer. Retrieved from   https://www.ncbi.nlm.nih.gov/pmc/articles/ PMC3595327/

Pan, S. Y., Zhou, J., Gibbons, L., Canadian Cancer Registries Epidemiology Research Group [CCRERG], & et al. (2011, August 24). Antioxidants and Breast Cancer Risk A population-based case-control study in Canada. Retrieved from https://www.ncbi.nlm.nih.gov/pmc/ articles/PMC3224257/

Pitchakarn, P., Chewonarin, T., Ogawa, K., & et al. (2013). Ellagic acid inhibits migration and invasion by prostate cancer cell lines. Retrieved from https://www.ncbi.nlm. nih.gov/pubmed/23803044

Pop, E. A., Fischer, L. M., & Coan, A. D. (2008). Effects of a high daily dose of soy isoflavones on DNA damage, apoptosis, and estrogenic outcomes in healthy postmenopausal women: a phase I clinical trial. Retrieved from https:// www.ncbi.nlm.nih.gov/pmc/articles/PMC2574732/

Prasad, A. S., Beck, F. W. J., Snell, D. C., & Kucuk, O. (2009). Zinc in cancer prevention. Retrieved from https://www. ncbi.nlm.nih.gov/pubmed/20155630

Raffaghello, L., Safdie, F., Bianchi, G., & et al. (2010). Fasting and differential chemotherapy protection in patients. Cell Cycle, 9(22), 4474–4476. doi: 10.4161/cc.9.22.13954

Rahman, I., & MacNee, W. (2000, September). Oxidative stress and regulation of glutathione in lung inflammation. Retrieved from https://www.ncbi.nlm.nih.gov/ pubmed/11028671

Rappaport, J. (n.d.). Changes in Dietary Iodine Explains Increasing Incidence of Breast Cancer with Distant Involvement in Young Women. Retrieved from https:// www.jcancer.org/v08p0174.htm

RGCC Group. (n.d.). Retrieved from https://www.rgcc-group.

com/

Rodriguez, B. D., & Palinski-Wade, E. (n.d.). The Lowdown on Glycemic Load - Diet and Nutrition Center. Retrieved from https://www.everydayhealth.com/diet-nutrition/101/nutrition-basics/the-glycemic-load.aspx

Rose, S., Fernie, & Fernie. (2019, October 31). All-Natural Chest Vapor Rub Recipe. Retrieved from https://gardentherapy.ca/vicks-vapo-rub-recipe/

Roshan, M. H., Shing, Y. K., & Pace, N. P. (2019, July 16). Metformin as an adjuvant in breast cancer treatment. Retrieved from https://www.ncbi.nlm.nih.gov/pmc/articles/PMC6637843/

Safdie, F. M., Dorff, T., Quinn, D., & et al. (2009). Fasting and cancer treatment in humans: A case series report. Aging, 1(12), 988–1007. doi: 10.18632/aging.100114

Safdie, F., Brandhorst, S., Wei, M., & et al. (2012). Fasting Enhances the Response of Glioma to Chemo- and Radiotherapy. PLoS ONE, 7(9). doi: 10.1371/journal.pone.0044603

Schubert, W., Cullberg, G., Edgar, B., & Hedner, T. (2005, April 21). Inhibition of 17β-estradiol metabolism by grapefruit juice in ovariectomized women. Retrieved from https://www.sciencedirect.com/science/article/pii/0378512294900124

Shibata, S., Hayakawa, K., Egashira, Y., & Sanada, H. (2007, April). Hypocholesterolemic mechanism of Chlorella: Chlorella and its indigestible fraction enhance hepatic cholesterol catabolism through up-regulation of cholesterol 7alpha-hydroxylase in rats. Retrieved from https://www.ncbi.nlm.nih.gov/pubmed/17420587

Sieri, S., Agnoli, C., & Pala, V. (2017, August 29). Dietary glycemic index, glycemic load, and cancer risk: results from the EPIC-Italy study. Retrieved from https://www. ncbi.nlm.nih.gov/pubmed/28851931

Soheilifar, S., Bidgoli, M., Hooshyarfard, A., & et al. (2018, September). Effect of Oral Bromelain on Wound Healing, Pain, and Bleeding at Donor Site Following Free Gingival Grafting: A Clinical Trial. Retrieved from https://www. ncbi.nlm.nih.gov/pmc/articles/PMC6397736/

Stanford Health Care. (n.d.). Phytochemicals. Retrieved from https://stanfordhealthcare.org/medical-clinics/cancer-nutrition-services/reducing-cancer-risk/phytochemicals. html

Stavrou, G., & Kotzampassi, K. (2017). Gut microbiome, surgical complications and probiotics. Retrieved from https:// www.ncbi.nlm.nih.gov/pmc/articles/PMC5198246/

Subramani, & Ramadevi. (2017, April 3). Role of Growth Hormone in Breast Cancer. Retrieved from https:// academic.oup.com/endo/article/158/6/1543/3098660.

Sugarman, J. (2014, March 10). Are Mistletoe Extract Injections the Next Big Thing in Cancer Therapy? Retrieved from https://hub.jhu.edu/magazine/2014/spring/mistletoe-therapy-cancer/

Sun, Y., Wang, W., & Tong, Y. (2019, November 28). Berberine Inhibits Proliferative Ability of Breast Cancer Cells by Reducing Metadherin. Retrieved from https://www.ncbi. nlm.nih.gov/pubmed/31779025

Suzana, S., Cham, B. G., Ahmad Rohi, G., Mohd Rizal, R., & et al. (2009, March). Relationship between selenium and breast cancer: a case-control study in the Klang Valley. Retrieved from https://www.ncbi.nlm.nih.gov/ pubmed/19352569

Suárez-Arroyo, I. J., Loperena-Alvarez, Y., Rosario-Acevedo, R., & Martínez-Montemayor, M. M. (2017, March).

A Promising Adjuvant Treatment for Breast Cancer. Retrieved from https://www.ncbi.nlm.nih.gov/pmc/articles/PMC5533290/

The Genetics of Cancer. (n.d.). Retrieved from https://www.cancer.gov/about-cancer/causes-prevention/genetics

Tongue Diagnosis in Chinese Medicine. (2020, February 19). Retrieved from https://giovanni-maciocia.com/tongue-gallery/

Toxic and Essential Elements. (n.d.). Retrieved from https://www.doctorsdata.com/toxic-essential-elements/

University of Salford. (2017, March 8). Vitamin C effective in targeting cancer stem cells. Retrieved from https://www.sciencedaily.com/releases/2017/03/170308083940.htm

Varady, K. A., & Hellerstein, M. K. (2007). Alternate-day fasting and chronic disease prevention: a review of human and animal trials. The American Journal of Clinical Nutrition, 86(1), 7–13. doi: 10.1093/ajcn/86.1.7

Verma, P., Jahan, S., Kim, T. H., & Goyal, P. K. (2011, September). Management of Radiation Injuries by Panax ginseng Extract. Retrieved from https://www.ncbi.nlm.nih.gov/pmc/articles/PMC3659536/

Vermeulen, M., & Klöpping-Ketelaars Ineke W. A. A. (2008). Bioavailability and Kinetics of Sulforaphane in Humans after Consumption of Cooked versus Raw Broccoli. Journal of Agricultural and Food Chemistry, 56(22), 10505–10509. doi: 10.1021/jf801989e

Vieira, C., Evangelista, S., Cirillo, R., & et al. (2000). Effect of ricinoleic acid in acute and subchronic experimental models of inflammation. Retrieved from https://www.ncbi.nlm.nih.gov/pubmed/11200362

Vieira, C., Fetzer, S., Sauer, S. K., & et al. . (2001, August).

Pro- and anti-inflammatory actions of ricinoleic acid: similarities and differences with capsaicin. Retrieved from https://www.ncbi.nlm.nih.gov/pubmed/11534859

Vinceti, M., Filippini, T., Del Giovane, C., Dennert, G., & et al. (2018, January 29). Selenium for preventing cancer. Retrieved from https://www.ncbi.nlm.nih.gov/pubmed/29376219

Vyas, S., Zaganjor, E., & Haigis, M. C. (2016, July 28). Mitochondria and Cancer. Retrieved from https://www.ncbi.nlm.nih.gov/pmc/articles/PMC5036969/

Wang, J., Xiong, X., & Feng, B. (2013). Effect of crataegus usage in cardiovascular disease prevention: an evidence-based approach. Retrieved from https://www.ncbi.nlm.nih.gov/pmc/articles/PMC3891531/

Wang, J., Liu, Q., & Yang, Q. (2012, November). Radiosensitization effects of berberine on human breast cancer cells. Retrieved from https://www.ncbi.nlm.nih.gov/pubmed/22895634

Wang, R., Yang, L., Li, S., Ye, D., & et al. (2018, January 21). Quercetin Inhibits Breast Cancer Stem Cells via Downregulation of Aldehyde Dehydrogenase 1A1 (ALDH1A1), Chemokine Receptor Type 4 (CXCR4), Mucin 1 (MUC1), and Epithelial Cell Adhesion Molecule (EpCAM). Retrieved from https://www.ncbi.nlm.nih.gov/pmc/articles/PMC5788241/

Winters, N., & Kelley, J. H. (2017). The metabolic approach to cancer: integrating deep nutrition, the ketogenic diet, and nontoxic bio-individualized therapies. White River Junction, VT: Chelsea Green Publishing.

Wright, J. L., Plymate, S., Doria-Cameron, A., Bain, C., & et al. (2013). A study of caloric restriction versus standard diet in overweight men with newly diagnosed prostate cancer: A randomized controlled trial. The Prostate,

73(12), 1345–1351. doi: 10.1002/pros.22682

Yue, P., Zhang, F., Zhao, Y., & et al. (n.d.). Berberine Enhances Chemosensitivity and Induces Apoptosis Through Dose-orchestrated AMPK Signaling in Breast Cancer. Retrieved from https://www.jcancer.org/v08p1679

Zhao, L., Wang, T., Dong, J., & et al. (2018, January 31). Liver-stomach disharmony pattern: theoretical basis, identification and treatment. Retrieved from https://www.sciencedirect.com/science/article/pii/S2095754818300085

Zhou, R., Chen, H., Chen, J., & et al. (2018, March 9). Extract from Astragalus membranaceus inhibit breast cancer cells proliferation via PI3K/AKT/mTOR signaling pathway. Retrieved from https://www.ncbi.nlm.nih.gov/pubmed/29523109

Ziaei, S., & Halaby, R. (2017, April 7). Dietary Isoflavones and Breast Cancer Risk. Retrieved from https://www.ncbi.nlm.nih.gov/pmc/articles/PMC5590054/

Zolkipli-Cunningham, Z., & Falk, M. J. (2017). Clinical effects of chemical exposures on mitochondrial function. Toxicology, 391, 90–99. doi: 10.1016/j.tox.2017.07.009

Printed in Great Britain
by Amazon